The Power of Herbal Remedies and Natural Medicine

EASE STRESS, SUPPORT IMMUNITY & RESTORE BALANCE NATURALLY

SAGE WILDER

ECOHEAL PUBLISHING

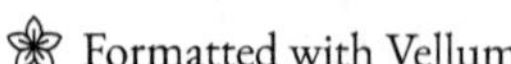 Formatted with Vellum

Contents

Introduction

Since I can recall, my father would create herbal mixtures to soothe my irritated skin during eczema flare-ups. He also used nature's antibiotics, honey and garlic, to help ease my colds. As an adult, I discovered the benefits of naturopathy. I adjusted my diet while incorporating supplements like Omega 3 and 6 for my eczema and prebiotics for my IBS. This experience inspired me to enrol in a course in Natural Medicine. Despite initial scepticism about the syllabus and fitting it into my busy schedule, I ultimately decided to advance my career in Biochemical Engineering instead. This sparked my passion for herbal remedies, forever transforming my approach to health and wellness.

This book is rooted in a simple yet powerful thesis: Herbal remedies offer a potent, accessible, and sustainable path to wellness. Through these pages, I invite you to discover how natural solutions can enhance your health and align you with a more sustainable way of living. Here, you will find remedies and a new health perspective that respects ancient traditions and modern science.

You're embarking on a comprehensive guide with practical advice on safely and effectively utilising herbs. This book covers all bases, from detailed step-by-step instructions for creating your tinctures and oils to precautions that ensure you use these remedies safely. I integrate wisdom from diverse traditions such as Ayurveda, Traditional Chinese Medicine, and Western herbalism, providing a well-rounded approach to herbal medicine.

I began my journey into the therapeutic powers of plants over a decade ago, fuelled by personal experiences and rigorous research. This path has shown me the effectiveness of herbal remedies and their potential to foster a deeper connection with the natural world. By choosing this book, you trust a guide who has navigated the vast landscape of natural medicine to distil only the most impactful practices and insights.

This narrative is open to blending time-honoured herbal traditions with cutting-edge scientific research. Every remedy and practice suggested herein is backed by scientific studies that underscore their efficacy, ensuring you receive trustworthy and transformative information.

Designed with you in mind—whether you're a health-conscious individual, an environmentally aware consumer, an older adult, a parent of young children, or someone managing chronic health issues—this book speaks directly to your needs and aspirations. It promises to enhance your health and elevate your entire approach to living well.

By integrating the practices outlined in this book, you stand to improve your immunity, prolong your life, and achieve a state of wellness that permeates every aspect of your being. It would help if you approached this book as a reader and actively participated in your health journey. Keep an open mind, experiment with the remedies, and embrace herbal medicine as a series of treatments and a lifestyle.

As we close this introduction, I share a message of hope and healing. The journey you are about to undertake has the potential to enrich your life, just as it has profoundly enriched mine. May the following pages inform you and inspire a deeper, more vibrant connection with health and well-being.

Welcome to a new chapter in your life, one scented with the healing power of herbs and paved with the wisdom of nature. Let's begin.

CHAPTER 1

Understanding Herbal Medicine

When I first delved into natural health, I was struck by the sharp contrast between modern pharmacies' sterile, clinical atmosphere and the lively, earthy ambience of an herbalist's workshop. The shelves lined with jars of dried herbs and the subtle scents of flowers and roots were a world apart. My curiosity was piqued when I learned that many of these plants had been used for thousands of years, carrying stories of ancient wisdom and healing. This realization inspired me to delve deeper into herbal medicine's history and cultural significance. It led me to appreciate its rich past and its potential to integrate seamlessly into contemporary healthcare practices.

THE EVOLUTION OF HERBAL MEDICINE FROM ANCIENT TO MODERN TIMES

Historical Progression

The journey of herbal medicine, a global phenomenon, is as old as civilization. Ancient Egyptians, for instance, utilized garlic and opium poppies, which were documented in the Ebers Papyrus around 1550 BCE. In ancient China, the Shennong Bencao Jing, a medicinal book from the 3rd century BCE, lists hundreds of medicinal plants and their uses, many of which are still used today. Like a global current, this knowledge travelled through cultures and continents, influenced by the Greeks and Romans before spreading throughout the Middle East and Europe during the Middle Ages. Each civilization utilized local plants for healing and added layers of medical knowledge and practice, contributing to a rich tapestry of global herbal medicine traditions.

The integration of these ancient practices into contemporary healthcare varies significantly by region. In some parts of the world, herbal remedies are as respected as modern pharmaceuticals, often used in tandem to treat illness and maintain health. For instance, in Germany, doctors commonly prescribe St. John's Wort for depression, and it is regulated and sold as a prescription medication. This acceptance and integration signify a respect for the plant's efficacy, grounded in centuries of use and increasingly supported by modern research.

Cultural Significance

Every culture has a unique relationship with the plants that grow around them, and understanding these relationships provides deeper insights into those communities' values and health practices. For example, Ayurveda and Traditional Chinese Medicine (TCM) use herbs to cure ailments, balance the body's energies and promote a harmonious life. These practices show a holistic approach to health, where the physical, spiritual, and emotional aspects are treated. This holistic view is gaining traction in the West, where the biomedical model traditionally focuses more narrowly on symptoms and single causative factors.

. . .

Regulatory Evolution

In the last century, the regulation of herbal medicine has evolved significantly. Herbal remedies have gained attention from medical institutions and regulatory bodies. The Dietary Supplement Health and Education Act of 1994 in the United States permitted herbal medicines to be marketed as dietary supplements without requiring FDA approval for safety and efficacy. However, this regulatory framework presents challenges and opportunities, emphasizing the need for consumer education to navigate the market safely.

Resurgence and Popularity

In recent decades, there has been a remarkable resurgence in the popularity of herbal medicine. This can be attributed to the increasing dissatisfaction with the side effects and limitations of conventional drugs and a broader movement towards more sustainable and environmentally friendly living practices. The appeal of reconnecting with nature and using remedies that have stood the test of time resonates with many people. The resurgence is also fuelled by a growing body of research that lends scientific credibility to many traditional uses of herbs and underscores their safety and efficacy. This trend towards natural and holistic health approaches shows no signs of waning, suggesting that herbal medicine will continue to play an essential role in global healthcare.

SCIENTIFIC BACKING OF HERBAL REMEDIES: SEPARATING FACT FROM FICTION

In my early days of exploring natural medicine, I was often met with scepticism. Friends, family, and healthcare professionals occasionally dismiss herbal remedies as folklore or placebo. This scepticism was reasonable, as herbal medicine contains its share of myths and unsubstantiated claims. However, over the years, a growing body of scientific research has begun to illuminate the true efficacy of many popular herbal remedies, providing a solid foundation for their use in modern healthcare. It's crucial for us, as advocates and users of herbal medicine, to understand and communicate this evidence-based perspective, ensuring that our choices are informed and effective.

The scientific validation of herbal remedies has seen significant advancements thanks to integrating modern research methodologies with traditional knowledge. Numerous studies now document the physiological effects of herbs, offering a clearer understanding of their mechanisms of action. For example, the anti-inflammatory properties of turmeric, primarily attributed to its curcumin content, have been well-documented in numerous clinical trials. These studies have shown that turmeric effectively reduces inflammation. This benefit aligns with its traditional use in Ayurvedic medicine to treat conditions like arthritis. Similarly, St. John's Wort, widely used in traditional practices for its antidepressant effects, has been extensively studied and is now recognized as an effective treatment for mild to moderate depression by the scientific community.

Despite these successes, the field of herbal medicine is also rife with misconceptions that can mislead consumers and harm the credibility of natural therapies. One common myth is that all-natural products are inherently safe. While many herbs are safe for most people when used appropriately, others can interact with medications or be toxic at high doses. It's essential to bust these myths by referencing scientific data, such as studies that outline the potential risks of herbs like kava, which has been linked to liver toxicity when misused. By debunking myths with evidence, we protect our health and enhance the legitimacy of herbal medicine.

Understanding how to evaluate the scientific literature on herbal remedies critically is another critical skill for anyone interested in natural health. Not all studies are created equal, and the quality of research can vary widely. When reviewing a survey, you should consider several factors, such as the study population size, the controls used, and whether the findings have been replicated. Peer-reviewed journals are generally reliable sources, but even then, it's wise to see if other studies have corroborated the results. For instance, while numerous studies support the efficacy of echinacea in boosting immune function, the results can vary based on the specific species of echinacea used, the part of the plant extracted, and the extraction methods employed, underscoring the need for careful analysis of the research.

While the body of evidence supporting herbal medicine continues to grow, there are still limitations in the research that need to be addressed. Many herbal studies need more funding, partly because plants cannot be patented like synthetic drugs, reducing the financial incentives for large-scale research. Additionally, the complexity of plant materials, which can contain hundreds of active compounds, makes it difficult to pinpoint which components are responsible for therapeutic effects. This complexity challenges the research process and highlights the vast potential for discovering new aspects of herbs that could enhance their application in medicine.

The potential of herbal medicine continues to expand as researchers delve deeper into the pharmacology of plants and as clinical trials become more sophisticated. With ongoing research, we can uncover more about the herbs we currently use and those that have yet to be fully explored. This ongoing evolution of knowledge enriches our understanding. It improves our ability to utilize these natural resources for health and healing. As we continue to advocate for and use herbal medicine, staying informed about the scientific underpinnings of our practices ensures that our approach remains credible and compelling.

ESSENTIAL HERBAL VOCABULARY: TERMS EVERY HERBALIST SHOULD KNOW

Navigating the world of herbal medicine can feel like learning a new language. Understanding the terminology is crucial for effective communication about the practices and benefits of herbal remedies. Knowing key terms enhances your understanding and application of herbal medicine, whether discussing remedies with healthcare professionals, researching plants, or reading labels on herbal products. Let's explore some fundamental vocabulary that forms the bedrock of the herbal lexicon, covering basic preparations, pharmacological terms, cultivation methods, and the therapeutic actions of herbs.

Basic Terminology

At the core of herbal medicine are terms that describe how herbs are prepared. A **_tincture_** is a concentrated herbal extract soaking a plant's bark, berries, leaves, or roots in alcohol or vinegar. The liquid extracts the plant's active compounds, resulting in a potent remedy that can be administered in small doses. **_Infusions_** and **_decoctions_** are both methods of removing the medicinal properties of herbs through water. However, they differ in technique and the parts of the plant for which they are best suited. Making an infusion, also called herbal tea, involves pouring boiling water over herbs and letting them steep. This method is perfect for extracting flavours and aromas from delicate plant parts like leaves and flowers. A **_decoction_** involves simmering tougher parts, such as roots or bark, to extract their essence. Finally, a **_salve_** is a thick, ointment-like preparation used topically. It combines infused oils with waxes or butters, which are heated and then cooled to form a protective barrier on the skin, aiding in healing and providing relief from various skin conditions.

. . .

Pharmacological Terms

Understanding the pharmacological aspects of herbs can significantly enhance your appreciation of their therapeutic potential. *Phytochemicals* are chemicals produced by plants that have biological activity in the human body. These can include nutrients and non-nutrient compounds contributing to the plant's colour, taste, and resistance to diseases and pests. *Alkaloids*, a class of phytochemicals, are nitrogen-containing compounds found in plants that often have potent effects on the human body; caffeine and morphine are well-known examples. *Flavonoids* are another group of phytochemicals known for their antioxidant and anti-inflammatory properties. They give fruits and vegetables their vibrant colours and are also found abundantly in herbs.

Cultivation Term

For those interested in growing their herbs or understanding where their herbal remedies come from, terms related to cultivation are invaluable. *Biodynamic* farming is an advanced form of organic farming that uses holistic regenerative practices, integrating plants, animals, and soil health and considering the influences of the lunar and cosmic cycles. *Permaculture* is another sustainable method of cultivation that mimics the natural ecosystem to create a self-sustaining environment. It emphasizes the use of native plants, which include many medicinal herbs. It aims to develop agricultural systems that are harmonious with their natural surroundings.

Therapeutic Action Terms

We use terms that categorize their therapeutic actions to describe how herbs act within the body. An *adaptogen* is a herb that helps the body resist physical, chemical, or biological stressors, supporting overall health and energy levels. *Antimicrobial* herbs can inhibit the growth of or destroy microorganisms, making them invaluable in fighting infections. ***Analgesic*** herbs relieve pain without causing loss of consciousness; willow bark, for instance, has been used for centuries as a natural analgesic.

Understanding these terms enriches your knowledge and empowers you to use herbal remedies more effectively and communicate more confidently about your herbal practices. Whether you're a novice herbal enthusiast or a seasoned practitioner, this foundational vocabulary is crucial in fostering a deeper connection with herbal medicine and enhancing your ability to care for yourself and others using the gifts of nature.

SAFETY FIRST: RECOGNIZING AND MANAGING RISKS WITH HERBAL MEDICINE

Navigating the world of herbal medicine requires understanding how to use herbs and awareness of their safety profiles. This knowledge is crucial, empowering you to make informed decisions and use herbal remedies effectively and safely. Let's start by addressing how to recognize high-quality, uncontaminated herbal products—a fundamental step in ensuring the efficacy and safety of your herbal treatments.

Selecting high-quality herbs is akin to choosing fresh produce. You want herbs that are vibrant, aromatic, and free from mould and decay. When sourcing dried herbs, look for colours as close as possible to the plant's natural state when fresh; dull, lifeless herbs may indicate poor storage conditions or age, which can diminish their therapeutic properties. The scent of the herbs should be solid and transparent, not musty or stale. If purchasing whole herbs, such as roots or leaves, ensure they are clean and free from any signs of insect damage or pollution. This attention to quality should extend to packaged products. Opt for suppliers who provide clear information about the source, processing methods, and storage of the herbs, as transparency is often a good indicator of quality.

Understanding potential side effects and interactions with medications must be addressed. While herbal remedies are generally safe when used correctly, they can cause adverse reactions or interact negatively with pharmaceutical medicines. St. John's Wort, for example, helps treat mild depression but can disrupt the potency of certain prescribed medications like birth control pills and specific antidepressants. It's essential to consult healthcare professionals, ideally with a conventional and herbal medicine background, before combining herbal treatments with pharmaceuticals. They can provide guidance based on the latest research and clinical guidelines to ensure your safety.

Understanding contraindications is another critical aspect of using herbal remedies safely. Certain herbs should be avoided in specific conditions or by populations. For example, pregnant women are generally advised to avoid herbs like goldenseal and mugwort, which can stimulate uterine contractions and potentially lead to complications. Similarly, individuals with autoimmune diseases might need to steer clear of immune-stimulating herbs like echinacea to prevent exacerbating their symptoms. This knowledge is pivotal to avoiding adverse effects and maximizing herbal remedies' therapeutic benefits.

Managing interactions between herbal remedies and pharmaceutical medications is a complex but vital part of using herbs safely. Many herbs can alter the metabolism of drugs, either increasing or decreasing their effects, which can have severe implications for your health. For instance, spices like garlic and ginkgo can increase the risk of bleeding when taken with blood thinners such as warfarin. To manage these interactions effectively, always disclose your use of herbal remedies to your healthcare provider and maintain an open line of communication about any new symptoms or changes in your condition. It's also advisable to keep a diary of your herbal consumption, noting types, quantities, and any side effects experienced, which can be invaluable during medical consultations.

Regarding safe consumption practices, adhering to recommended dosages and durations of use is paramount. More is not always better in the realm of herbal medicine. For example, high doses of liquorice root over an extended period can lead to potassium depletion and high blood pressure. Each herb has its optimal dosage and duration of use, often determined by factors such as the specific condition being treated, the individual's age, and overall health. These guidelines are typically available in herbal reference books or from professional herbalists. They should always be followed to minimize risks

Lastly, a brief overview of the regulation of herbal products can help you make informed choices. In many countries, herbal products are regulated differently than pharmaceutical drugs, often classified as dietary supplements. This classification means that while manufacturers are responsible for ensuring the safety of their products, the products do not undergo the rigorous pre-market testing that drugs do. As a result, the quality and potency of herbal products can vary widely between brands and batches. To mitigate this, look for products certified by reputable third-party organizations, such as the U.S. Pharmacopeia (USP) or ConsumerLab. These certifications indicate that the product has been independently tested and meets specific standards for quality and safety.

By understanding these critical aspects of safety in herbal medicine, you can confidently incorporate herbal remedies into your healthcare regime. Remember, knowledge is not just power—it is protection. Armed with the correct information, you can harness the healing power of herbs while ensuring that your health journey remains safe and beneficial.

CHAPTER 2

Identifying and Sourcing Herbs

Connecting with nature is profoundly grounding, mainly through foraging for your herbs. Picture this: you're walking through a lush forest, the air is fresh with the scent of pine and earth, and beneath your feet, a carpet of greenery harbours treasures waiting to be discovered. Foraging isn't just about gathering herbs; it's a way to deepen your relationship with the environment and gain an intimate understanding of the natural resources surrounding us. We find herbs and a path to greater wellness and sustainability in the forest's whispers.

FORAGING FOR HERBS: A BEGINNER'S GUIDE TO WILDCRAFTING

Ethical Foraging

As you embark on your foraging journey, it's crucial to approach it with respect and responsibility. Ethical foraging ensures that our interactions with nature are sustainable and beneficial not just to us but also to the ecosystems from which we draw. Always adhere to the principle of taking no more than what you need, which is usually recommended as one-third of a patch of wild plants. This practice helps to preserve the plant populations and biodiversity of the area. Furthermore, be mindful of where you forage. Protected areas and private properties often have restrictions, and it's essential to respect these boundaries to support conservation efforts and maintain good relationships with landowners and local communities.

Safety in Identification

One of the fundamental skills in foraging is the ability to identify plants correctly. Misidentification can lead not only to ineffective remedies but also to potentially harmful consequences. Start with a good field guide specific to the area you are exploring. This guide provides detailed photographs and descriptions that help you distinguish between similar-looking plants. I recommend spending time with experienced foragers or participating in guided walks organized by local herbalists or naturalist groups. These experts can provide hands-on learning, and insights often must be captured in books. Additionally, familiarize yourself with the toxic plants in your region to ensure your foraging adventures remain safe.

The legality of foraging varies by region and land type. National parks and protected areas may have strict guidelines or prohibitions. Check local regulations and obtain permits to forage responsibly and support conservation efforts.

Starter Plants

For those new to foraging, starting with easy-to-identify and widely used plants can make the process more enjoyable and less daunting. Dandelion, for example, is a common herb easily identified by its distinctive yellow flower and rosette of jagged leaves. It's a versatile plant used for everything from herbal teas to salads, and it boasts a range of health benefits, including liver support and inflammation reduction. Another good starter plant is plantain, which often appears in lawns and has broad, ribbed leaves. It's excellent for making soothing salves for bug bites and skin irritations. Nettle, though it requires gloves to handle due to its stinging hairs, is another superb choice. Once processed, it can be used in soups, teas, and more, offering benefits such as allergy relief and iron supplementation.

Identifying Common Medicinal Plants

To help you begin your foraging journey, consider this visual aid —a simple chart of common medicinal plants, their identifying features, and their primary uses. This guide can be a handy reference for quick identification during your foraging expeditions.

Scan the QR code for the Common Medicinal Herb Chart or Click on the link to access the chart.

By embracing ethical foraging practices, safety in identification, adherence to legal guidelines, and starting with easily recognizable plants, you set the foundation for a rewarding and sustainable foraging practice. As you walk through nature, basket in hand, remember that each plant you gently harvest carries a story of ecological balance and human wellness—a legacy that you are now part of.

GROWING YOUR MEDICINAL HERB GARDEN

Creating a medicinal herb garden is like planting your living pharmacy, where each leaf and root offers unique healing properties. As you consider embarking on this rewarding endeavour, the initial step is selecting the right herbs. It's essential to choose plants that thrive in your local climate and fit well within your available space, whether a sprawling backyard or a modest balcony. Begin with versatile herbs like lavender, renowned for its calming properties and can grow well in various climates, from excellent to warm. It requires full sun and good drainage, making it suitable for garden beds and containers. Another great choice is chamomile, known for its soothing effects on the digestive system and nerves. It prefers more excellent conditions and can quickly be grown in pots or designated garden patches.

Moving beyond the selection of herbs, employing organic cultivation practices is crucial for maintaining the purity and potency of your medicinal plants. This means avoiding synthetic pesticides and fertilizers, which can leach unwanted chemicals into your herbs and, ultimately, into the remedies you create. Instead, organic compost should be used to enrich the soil, and natural pest control methods such as companion planting should be considered. For example, planting garlic near roses can help deter pests naturally without chemical interventions.

It's essential to plan your garden carefully, as the layout can significantly impact the health and productivity of your medicinal plants. First, consider the specific needs of each herb, such as sunlight, water, and soil quality. For example, mint can spread rapidly, so it's best to plant it in containers to prevent it from taking over. On the other hand, echinacea needs deep soil, so it's better to plant it directly in garden beds with plenty of space to grow. Sketch out your garden layout, placing each herb where it can thrive based on its natural requirements. This careful planning will help your herbs flourish and make it easier to maintain your garden.

Finally, the true magic of a medicinal herb garden is its ability to transform these plants into remedies that can enhance your health and well-being. The possibilities are endless, from simple teas and tinctures to more complex salves and syrups. Creating these remedies begins with harvesting, a mindful practice that involves selecting the right plant parts at the right time for optimal potency. For instance, harvesting leaves and flowers in the morning after the dew has evaporated but before the sun is high ensures they are at their peak medicinal quality. Once harvested, the herbs can be used fresh or dried and stored throughout the year. This direct connection from seed to remedy deepens your relationship with the healing power of nature but also empowers you to take charge of your health in the most natural way possible.

ETHICAL AND SUSTAINABLE SOURCING OF HERBS

In our quest for wellness, it's vital to consider the efficacy of the herbal remedies we choose and the impact of their sourcing on the environment and communities. Selecting suppliers prioritizing ethical and sustainable practices is crucial in ensuring that our health remedies do not come at the earth's or its inhabitants' expense. Ethical sourcing involves selecting herbs from suppliers who responsibly harvest resources, ensuring their methods support the environment and the local communities' social structures. This approach often includes adhering to standards that prevent over-harvesting and promote fair worker compensation.

Prioritize suppliers who adhere to certified organic and fair-trade practices to ensure the herbs you buy are grown without harmful pesticides and herbicides and that farmers and workers are paid fair wages and work under safe conditions. This helps build sustainable communities and supports environmental conservation efforts.

Supporting local herbal businesses adds another layer of sustainability to your practices by reducing the carbon footprint, contributing to the local economy, and promoting agricultural practices in tune with the regional ecosystem.

The importance of conservation-minded sourcing practices becomes particularly evident when dealing with herbs at risk of over-harvesting. Many popular herbs, such as wild ginseng and goldenseal, face threats from unsustainable harvesting practices that could lead to their disappearance from natural habitats by choosing suppliers who cultivate these herbs rather than harvest them from wild populations or who implement sustainable wild-harvesting practices that allow these plant populations to regenerate, you contribute to conserving vital medicinal resources. It is also beneficial to educate yourself about the herbs considered endangered or vulnerable, which can be found through resources like the United Plant Savers' "At-Risk" list, a tool that helps herbalists and consumers make informed decisions about the herbs they use and promote.

Developing solid relationships with your herb suppliers can improve the quality and sustainability of your herbal products. Knowing your suppliers personally provides insights into their harvesting, production, and distribution processes, which can help you make better decisions. These relationships also facilitate the open and transparent exchange of information. You can communicate your preferences for sustainable practices and ethically sourced products, and suppliers can offer assurances of their commitment to these standards. Suppliers are often enthusiastic about sharing their knowledge and practices with genuinely interested consumers, leading to a mutually beneficial relationship that supports ethical herbalism principles.

. . .

By embracing these practices, you ensure your wellness aligns with the broader principles of environmental stewardship and social responsibility. This holistic approach enhances your health and contributes to the planet's and its communities' health, creating a sustainable cycle of wellness that extends beyond individual benefits. As you continue to explore the vast world of herbal medicine, let these principles guide your choices, enriching your practice with a deep sense of purpose and integrity.

STORING HERBS FOR POTENCY: BEST PRACTICES

When you've taken the time to select, forage, or cultivate your herbs carefully, proper storage becomes the crucial next step to ensure they retain their healing properties and remain safe for use. Think of each jar of dried herbs as a capsule of nature's magic, holding potential relief and wellness within. Preserving the potency of these herbs hinges on understanding and managing a few critical factors of storage: conditions, shelf life, organization, and contamination prevention.

Storage Conditions

To maintain the therapeutic efficacy of dried herbs, store them in a cool, dark, and dry place to avoid the degradation of active compounds. Glass jars with airtight seals are best used to prevent moisture and mould growth. If using clear jars, store them in a dark place or wrap them to block light and preserve the herbs' colour and essential oils.

Shelf Life

The shelf life of dried herbs varies depending on the herb and storage conditions. Leafy herbs and flowers can stay potent for 1-2 years if stored correctly. Roots and barks can be kept for up to 3 years. Check the colour, smell, and texture to test potency. Label herbs with purchase or harvest dates for easier management. To maintain the therapeutic efficacy of dried herbs, store them in a cool, dark, and dry place to avoid the degradation of active compounds.

Labelling and Organization

Labelling and organizing stored herbs for easy access and safety is essential. Label each container with the herb's name, harvest or purchase date, and additional notes. This is crucial for similar-looking herbs to avoid mix-ups. Organize them alphabetically or by category (culinary, medicinal, topical) for efficient use.

Preventing Contamination

Protecting dried herbs from contamination is crucial for safety and efficacy. Always use clean, dry utensils and sterilized containers when storing and transferring herbs. Clean containers thoroughly between uses to avoid cross-contamination. Proper herb storage enhances the longevity and effectiveness of your herbal remedies, reflecting a dedication to a sustainable, health-conscious lifestyle. This also applies to any tinctures or salves made at home.

As we conclude this chapter on identifying and sourcing herbs, we've explored how to ethically forage, cultivate, and store your herbal bounty. These practices deepen your connection to the natural world and empower you to maintain and enhance your health independently. With your herbs safely stored and ready for use, we transition into the next chapter, where we will delve into the art of preparing these herbs into effective remedies. Here, the true magic of herbal medicine comes to life as we transform raw plant materials into healing concoctions that can soothe, invigorate, and restore.

CHAPTER 3

Preparation Methods and Tools

Imagine yourself in a serene kitchen, surrounded by jars of dried herbs and the gentle hum of a simmering pot, as you embark on the artful practice of creating herbal preparations. This chapter is designed to transform that vivid image into your daily reality. Here, you will learn to master the craft of making herbal teas, decoctions, and infusions—each a gateway to accessing herbs' profound wellness benefits. These methods are not just procedures; they are rituals that connect us more deeply with the healing powers of nature. By understanding the nuances of these practices, you equip yourself with the knowledge to nurture your health and that of your loved ones.

MAKING HERBAL TEAS, DECOCTIONS, AND INFUSIONS

Differences and Uses

The world of herbal liquid preparations is rich and varied, with each type offering unique benefits and suited for specific uses. The most familiar herbal teas are made by steeping herbs in hot water.

This method is ideal for extracting the full medicinal benefits from delicate plant parts like leaves and flowers, as they release their valuable properties at lower temperatures. Teas are perfect for quick preparation and are best enjoyed soon after brewing to maximize their flavour and therapeutic benefits.

Decoctions involve simmering more challenging plant materials, like roots, bark, and seeds, which require more time and heat to extract their active compounds. This method is perfect for extracting deep-seated nutrients. Herbalists often use it to target more chronic conditions or when they need a more potent dose.

Infusions are similar to teas but involve a longer steeping time. Herbalists often use them for the most fragile plant parts, such as petals or delicate leaves. Cold or room-temperature water is sometimes used instead of hot water to preserve sensitive oils and compounds that heat might damage. Infusions are excellent for creating potent medicinal drinks that harness herbs' gentle yet powerful qualities.

Step-by-Step Guidance

Creating these herbal preparations is both an art and a science. To make a herbal tea:

1. Begin by boiling water and pouring it over the herb, usually about one teaspoon of dried herb per cup of water.
2. Cover the vessel to prevent the escape of aromatic compounds and steep for about 10-15 minutes.
3. Strain and enjoy the tea, perhaps with a touch of honey or lemon for flavour.
4. Place your more rigid materials, like burdock root or cinnamon bark, in a pot with cold water for a decoction.
5. Use about one tablespoon of dried herb per cup of water

6. Slowly bring the mixture to a boil, then reduce the heat and simmer gently for 20-30 minutes, covered.
7. Strain the liquid, and you can drink it immediately or store it in the refrigerator for up to 48 hours.

When making an infusion, take one ounce of dried or two ounces of fresh herbs, place them in a jar, and cover them with boiling water. Use about one pint of water per ounce of dried herbs. Cover the jar to keep the heat in and steep for 30-45 minutes or even longer for a more potent infusion—strain and sip throughout the day.

Tools of the Trade

The tools required for these preparations are simple and likely already in your kitchen. An essential set of tools includes a stainless-steel pot for decoctions, a glass or ceramic teapot or jar for infusions, and a strainer or cheesecloth for separating the liquid from the plant material. A dedicated set of tools for your herbal crafting can enhance the experience and keep your preparations clean and organized.

Maximizing Efficacy

To maximize the benefits of your herbal preparations, consider the timing of your harvest, the source of your water, and the duration of your steeping. Herbs are most potent when harvested at the right time of year and time of day. After the dew has evaporated, early morning is ideal for picking leaves and flowers. Using spring or filtered water can also enhance the purity of your teas, decoctions, and infusions, as tap water may contain chemicals that alter the taste and medicinal qualities of the herbs. Lastly, be mindful of steeping times—too short may not extract the full benefit of the herbs, while too long can produce a bitter taste.

Create delightful, healing beverages that soothe the mind and nurture the body. Each sip carries the essence of the earth, a reminder of the natural world's wisdom and generosity. Reflect on this connection and enjoy the peace and wellness that comes from within.

THE ART OF CRAFTING TINCTURES AND EXTRACTS

Tinctures are a cornerstone of herbal medicine, offering a potent and convenient way to extract and preserve herbs' medicinal properties. These liquid extracts are effective and long-lasting, making them a practical addition to your natural medicine cabinet. Let's explore the foundational aspects of making herbal tinctures. This process marries the ancient art of herbalism with modern-day precision and understanding.

Tincture-making begins with selecting the appropriate solvent, which is crucial as it determines the extraction efficiency and the type of compounds extracted from the herbs. The most used solvent is *alcohol* because it can dissolve many plant constituents, including alkaloids, terpenes, and flavonoids. Alcohol also acts as a preservative, allowing the tincture to remain potent and stable for years. When choosing alcohol, aim for a proof of 80 to 100, typically found in vodka or brandy, which provides an ideal balance of water and alcohol to extract both water-soluble and alcohol-soluble compounds.

For those who prefer a non-alcoholic option, glycerine is a suitable alternative. *Glycerine* tinctures, often called glycerites, are sweeter and thicker than alcohol-based tinctures, making them particularly palatable for children. While glycerine is effective for extracting flavours and nutrients, it is not as potent as alcohol in extracting certain therapeutic compounds, which may limit the efficacy of some glycerites compared to their alcoholic counterparts. Another alternative is *vinegar*, a good choice for removing minerals from herbs and an excellent medium for those looking for a food-based solvent. However, vinegar tinctures typically have a shorter shelf life than those made with alcohol.

The process of making a tincture typically involves maceration or percolation. ***Maceration*** is the more common method, where dried or fresh herbs are chopped and then soaked in your solvent of choice in a sealed jar. The jar is kept in a cool, dark place, and the mixture is shaken daily to encourage extraction. After a period ranging from two to six weeks, depending on the herb and desired strength, the mixture is strained, and the liquid is bottled. Percolation, conversely, is a quicker method that involves passing your solvent through a column of finely chopped herbs, collecting the tincture as it drips out of the bottom. This method requires specific equipment and a more precise setup. However, it can produce a tincture in just a day or two, with often a stronger concentration than maceration.

Storing and using tinctures properly is crucial for maintaining their potency and therapeutic effectiveness. Tinctures should be stored in dark glass bottles in a cool, dark place to protect them from light and heat, which can degrade the active compounds over time. Amber or cobalt blue bottles are ideal as they filter out harmful UV rays. Label each bottle with the herb name, type of solvent, concentration, and the date of preparation, which helps track their potency and lifespan.

When it comes to using tinctures, the dosage varies depending on the strength of the tincture, the nature of the herb, and the individual's age, weight, and health condition. Generally, the tincture dosage is small, typically ranging from a few drops to a couple of millilitres, taken two to three times a day. It is essential to start with a lower dose and adjust as needed based on the effects and your body's response. Tinctures can be taken directly under the tongue for fast absorption into the bloodstream or added to a small amount of water or tea. For chronic conditions or general wellness, tinctures can be used consistently over time, while acute symptoms can be used as needed for relief.

. . .

By mastering the art of tincture making, you expand your toolkit for natural health care and connect with a tradition that has supported wellness for generations. Whether you choose alcohol, glycerine, or vinegar as your solvent, and whether you opt for maceration or percolation, the tinctures you create will carry the concentrated essence of the plants, ready to support your health whenever needed.

CREATING HERBAL OILS AND SALVES FOR TOPICAL USE

The creation of herbal oils and salves combines the simplicity of traditional methods with the profound potency of nature's offerings. As you embark on this path, imagine transforming the vibrant essence of herbs into soothing, healing concoctions that can be applied to the skin, nurturing it with the purity of natural ingredients. Let's explore the delicate process of infusing oils with medicinal herbs. This practice lets you capture plants' therapeutic properties in a versatile and profoundly comforting form.

Infusing oils involves gently coaxing the active compounds from herbs into a carrier oil. You can achieve this process through heat or time. Begin by selecting your herbs—both fresh and dried can be used, though each has its nuances. Dry fresh herbs slightly to minimize water content and prevent spoilage. Herbs like calendula, lavender, and chamomile are excellent choices due to their skin-soothing properties. Place the herbs in a clean, dry jar, then pour a carrier oil over them until fully submerged. The choice of oil is significant; oils like olive, jojoba, or sweet almonds are excellent for the skin and have a stable shelf life.

For a heat infusion, you can use a double boiler to gently warm the oil and herbs over low heat, careful not to let it boil, to protect the delicate properties of the oil. Typically, this process takes about 1-

2 hours. Alternatively, for those who prefer a slower, more traditional method, the solar infusion method harnesses the power of sunlight. Place the jar in a sunny spot and let the sun's natural warmth facilitate the infusion over two to three weeks. Whichever method you choose, once the infusion process is complete, strain the herbs from the oil using cheesecloth. What remains is a richly infused oil that carries the essence and benefits of the herbs.

Transitioning from oil to salve involves a few more steps but is equally rewarding. To make an essential herbal salve:

1. Take your infused oil and gently warm it in a double boiler.
2. Add about a quarter cup of beeswax for every oil cup, which acts as a thickening agent.
3. Stir continuously until the beeswax is completely melted and combined with the oil.
4. Add essential oils for additional therapeutic benefits and aroma; lavender or tea tree oil are popular for their soothing and antiseptic properties.
5. Once thoroughly mixed, pour the mixture into clean tins or glass jars and allow it to cool and solidify.
6. Once cooled, it will transform into a smooth, spreadable balm, perfect for addressing dry skin, minor cuts, or abrasions.

The choice of carrier oil in your infusions and salves can significantly affect the final product's texture, absorption rate, and shelf life. When selecting a carrier oil, consider the specific needs of your skin type and the therapeutic properties you desire. For example, **coconut oil** is highly moisturizing. It has inherent antibacterial properties, making it an excellent choice for treating dry or irritated skin. In contrast, grapeseed oil is lighter and has astringent qualities, ideal for oily or acne-prone skin. ***Jojoba oil*** is a perfect choice for various skin types as it resembles natural oils. Its versatility makes it an excellent option for different skincare needs but it is the most expensive. My choice of oil is coconut, although, at room temperature, it is solid due to its higher melting point. Carrying out a patch test before topically applying any of these oils is essential. Understanding these oil properties allows you to tailor your herbal oils and salves to suit specific conditions and preferences, enhancing their effectiveness and personalization.

Proper packaging and labelling are crucial, especially if you plan to gift or sell your herbal oils and salves. Not only do they ensure the product's integrity by protecting it from light and air exposure, but they also provide essential information about the contents. Use amber or cobalt blue glass containers to shield the products from light, which can degrade the oils over time. Labels should clearly state the ingredients, the date of production, and any usage instructions or warnings. This attention to detail elevates the perceived value of your herbal products. It ensures that they are used safely and effectively.

When you create your herbal oils and salves, you engage in a process that nurtures both the spirit and the body. Every step, from selecting the herbs to packaging the final product, is filled with intention and care, reflecting a dedication to natural health and sustainability. These preparations are not just surface-level treatments; they are tangible representations of holistic wellness made by your hands and infused with the healing power of the natural world. Whether you use them to soothe a child's scraped knee or alleviate skin issues, these herbal mixtures provide gentle, effective care while deepening your connection to the earth and its healing resources.

THE ESSENTIALS OF HERBAL MEDICINE KIT: TOOLS AND CONTAINERS

Embarking on the path of home herbalism is akin to setting up a personal wellness sanctuary where each tool and container plays a crucial role in crafting remedies that nurture and heal. As you curate your herbal medicine kit, consider it an extension of your care and respect for the healing powers of nature. It's not merely about having the right tools; it's about creating a space that inspires and supports your herbal practice.

The foundation of a well-equipped herbal medicine kit starts with a few essential tools. A mortar and pestle, made from ceramic, glass, or stone, is indispensable for grinding and blending herbs, allowing you to unlock their full medicinal potential. Precision scales are crucial for measuring herbs and other ingredients, ensuring recipe accuracy. This is especially important when working with potent herbs where dosages need to be exact. A set of stainless-steel funnels of various sizes will aid in transferring liquids without spillage, maintaining cleanliness and efficiency in your preparations.

Additionally, having a selection of spoons and spatulas, preferably in stainless steel or bamboo, is beneficial for stirring and scooping. These tools serve their functional purposes and connect you to the tactile experience of creating, which is at the heart of herbalism.

When selecting containers for storing your herbal creations, choosing the suitable materials, sizes, and seals is vital to preserving the quality and efficacy of your remedies. Glass is often the best choice for storage as it doesn't react with herbs or oils and can be easily sterilized. Amber glass is precious as it protects contents from ultraviolet light, which can degrade many herbs over time. Small, wide-mouthed jars are practical for creams, salves, and powders, allowing easy access and preventing waste. Bottles with droppers are ideal for tinctures and extracts, offering convenience and precision when administering doses. Ensure that all containers have tight-fitting lids to avoid exposure to air, which can also diminish the potency of herbal preparations.

Maintaining your herbal medicine kit involves regular care to ensure your tools and containers remain clean, organized, and ready for use. Always clean tools immediately after use, using hot water and natural soap, and dry them thoroughly to prevent rust or mould. Containers should be sterilized before each use, which can be done by boiling them in water or using a natural sanitizer. This ensures the purity of your remedies and extends the life of your tools and containers. Keeping your kit organized can save you time and enhance your efficiency. Designate specific areas or containers for different tools and supplies, and label everything clearly. This not only helps in quickly finding what you need but also prevents cross-contamination.

For those looking to expand their herbal medicine practices, consider adding specialized tools that align with your interests and needs. A high-quality blender or grinder can be invaluable for creating fine powders or smooth pastes from tough herbs and roots. For those interested in distillation, a small still can be an excellent tool for creating essential oils and hydrosols at home. Advanced measuring tools like a refractometer, which measures the concentration of aqueous solutions, can be helpful for those making intricate herbal extracts and tinctures. These tools open new possibilities in your herbal practice, allowing you to explore and create more deeply and precisely.

As you assemble and care for your herbal medicine kit, remember that each item is vital to your journey toward natural wellness. These tools and containers are not just practical aids; they are vessels of transformation that turn raw plants into healing remedies. They hold the potential to soothe, heal, and rejuvenate, bridging the gap between nature's wild potency and the comforting sanctuary of your home.

This chapter explores the foundational elements of creating and maintaining an effective herbal medicine kit. From selecting the right tools and containers to understanding the best practices for care and organization, these insights help solidify your practice of home herbalism. As you continue to grow in your herbal journey, these tools will assist in crafting effective remedies and deepen your connection to the healing traditions that have nurtured humanity for centuries.

Looking ahead, the next chapter will guide you through the diverse and enriching world of herbal remedies for digestive health, where you will learn how to harness the gentle yet powerful benefits of herbs to nourish and balance your digestive system.

CHAPTER 4

Herbal Remedies for Digestive Health

As we navigate through the bustling rhythms of our daily lives, our digestive health often takes a backseat until discomfort arises, reminding us of its pivotal role in our overall well-being. Think of your digestive system as a bustling city where everything needs to flow smoothly for harmony and health to prevail. When traffic jams occur in the form of cramps, bloating, or nausea, herbal teas emerge as gentle, effective conductors, guiding the chaotic energy of digestive distress back to a calm efficiency. This chapter delves into the art of using herbal teas—a practice as ancient as it is soothing—to address common digestive discomforts, offering you a natural pathway to maintaining digestive harmony.

SOOTHING TEAS FOR DIGESTIVE DISCOMFORT

In the world of herbal remedies, teas hold a special place, particularly when addressing the delicate balance of digestive health. Simple to prepare and enjoyable to consume, herbal teas blend the therapeutic grace of nature with the comforting warmth of a familiar ritual. Let's explore some of the most revered natural antispasmodics. These are drugs that relieve or prevent spasms of the smooth muscles, such as the stomach and intestine. Examples include peppermint, chamomile, and ginger. Each is a powerhouse, capable of easing cramps and spasms that can disrupt your day.

Natural Antispasmodics: The Gentle Power of Peppermint, Chamomile, and Ginger

Peppermint is not just a flavour for candies; it is a potent antispasmodic that relaxes the smooth muscles of the digestive tract. This can ease the painful spasms that accompany conditions like irritable bowel syndrome (IBS). Peppermint tea is often used in herbal remedies for digestive problems due to its quick relief of stomach issues.

Chamomile, with its gentle floral essence, is a balm for the nervous and digestive systems alike. It soothes the mind and muscles lining the stomach and intestines, reducing cramping and inflammation. Whether dealing with stress-related digestive issues or a simple case of indigestion, chamomile tea is a gentle healer, restoring peace to your internal landscape.

Ginger, a root celebrated across various cultures for its medicinal properties, offers dual benefits for digestive health. It is particularly revered for its ability to alleviate nausea and stimulate digestion. A warm cup of ginger tea can help settle an upset stomach, making it a favoured remedy for morning sickness, motion sickness, and food-related discomfort. Its warming properties stimulate digestive enzymes, enhancing the body's digestive capabilities and ensuring nutrients are absorbed efficiently.

Fennel's Bloat Relief: A Carminative Champion

Fennel seeds are more than just antispasmodics. They act as a carminative, relieving bloating and gas. The sweet, liquorice-like flavour of fennel is pleasant in teas. It helps relax the digestive tract, dissipating trapped gas and comforting a bloated belly. Enjoying fennel tea after meals can be an effective way to maintain digestive comfort.

Herbal Blends for IBS: Tailored Comfort for Chronic Conditions

For those managing chronic gastrointestinal disorders such as IBS, the strategic blending of herbs can amplify the soothing effects of individual plants. Consider a tea blend that combines peppermint's antispasmodic powers with chamomile's calming effects and the digestive support of ginger. This trio, when brewed together, can significantly alleviate the chronic symptoms of IBS, offering a holistic approach to managing the condition. The ritual of preparing and sipping this herbal blend can also provide psychological comfort, reminding you that relief is within your grasp.

Creating Your Healing Tea Blend

To assist you in crafting your digestive tea blends, consider this simple visual guide:

1. **Select Your Base Herb**: Choose one primary herb that targets your main symptom, such as peppermint for spasms.
2. **Add Supportive Herbs**: Incorporate one or two herbs that complement the base in flavour and function, like ginger for nausea.
3. **Measure and Mix**: Use one teaspoon of each dried herb per cup of boiling water.

4. **Brew with Care**: To preserve the essential oils, steep your blend for 5-10 minutes, covered.
5. **Enjoy and Observe**: Sip the tea slowly and note its effects on your symptoms.

This guide helps create effective blends and empowers you to tweak them according to your specific needs and preferences, making each cup a personalized healing experience.

In exploring herbal teas for digestive health, we traversed from the soothing realms of peppermint, chamomile, and ginger to the comforting embrace of fennel, illustrating how we can harness nature's bounty to support our digestive well-being. As you integrate these teas into your life, may they offer you physical relief and a moment of peace, a reminder of herbal remedies' gentle yet profound power. Whether seeking immediate relief from a meal gone awry or managing a chronic condition, these herbal teas stand ready to soothe and restore, cup by comforting cup.

NATURAL SOLUTIONS FOR CONSTIPATION RELIEF

Many people shy away from openly discussing constipation, but it significantly impacts quality of life. While over-the-counter medications often treat it, an increasing number of people are turning to more natural approaches to find relief. Certain herbs have proven especially beneficial due to their high fibre content and gentle laxative properties. By integrating these herbal solutions into our daily routines, we can enhance our digestive health naturally and effectively.

Herbs like **psyllium husk** and **flaxseed** are celebrated for their rich fibre content, making them excellent choices for easing constipation. Psyllium husk originates from the seeds of the Plantago Ovata plant and is highly potent. It absorbs water in the intestines, making bowel movements more accessible and manageable. Similarly, besides its omega-3 fatty acids, flaxseed contains soluble and insoluble fibre, which helps to bulk up stool and stimulate bowel movements. Integrating these herbs into your diet can be as simple as adding a tablespoon of ground flaxseed to your morning smoothie or mixing psyllium husk into a glass of water before meals. It's essential, however, to increase your intake gradually to give your digestive system time to adjust and to avoid potential bloating.

Hydration plays an indispensable role in the effectiveness of these fibre-rich herbs. Fibre can exacerbate constipation without adequate water, leading to further discomfort. When you increase your fibre intake through herbs, you should also increase your water consumption. This combination works synergistically to soften stool and enhance gut motility. Think of water as the transporter that helps fibre do its job more efficiently, moving waste smoothly through your digestive tract. Keeping a water bottle handy throughout the day or setting reminders to drink water can be effective strategies to ensure you stay well-hydrated.

While fibre-rich herbs and hydration form the foundation for natural constipation relief, a more direct approach is sometimes necessary, especially in severe or chronic constipation cases. This is where gentle laxatives such as senna and cascara sagrada come into play. **Senna**, used for centuries, contains compounds called Sennosides that irritate the lining of the bowel, causing a laxative effect. Similarly, cascara sagrada contains substances that stimulate the colon. However, you should use these herbs with caution. They are powerful, and their overuse can lead to dependency or disrupt the natural tone of your bowel muscles. It's advisable to use these herbs under the guidance of a healthcare provider and only for short periods.

Incorporating these natural solutions into your routine should be approached holistically. Start your day with a glass of water mixed with flaxseed or psyllium to boost your digestive system. Include ample fluids throughout the day to support the process. If you're using senna or cascara sagrada, consider taking them in the evening, as they typically require several hours, ensuring that your body responds to them naturally overnight. This routine not only addresses constipation when it occurs but also works as a preventive measure, maintaining regularity and digestive health over time.

By understanding and utilizing these natural herbs and practices, you equip yourself to manage and improve your digestive health gently and effectively. Remember, the key is balance and moderation, listening to your body's responses, and adjusting your methods accordingly. Through these steps, you can enjoy the benefits of a well-functioning digestive system, enhancing your overall health and well-being.

BITTERS AND TONICS FOR HEALTHY DIGESTION

In the realm of natural digestive aids, bitters and tonics hold a special place, revered not only for their ability to alleviate immediate digestive complaints but also for their contributions to long-term digestive health. Bitters are fascinating; they are not merely substances that surprise our taste buds but are catalysts for better digestive health. When you taste something bitter, it signals your body to kickstart the production of digestive juices, enhancing your ability to break down food efficiently and absorb nutrients effectively. This natural reflex, often overlooked in our modern diet, which leans towards sweetness, is crucial for optimal digestive function.

The role of bitters extends beyond the initial bitter shock on your tongue. They stimulate the secretion of digestive enzymes and bile, promoting the thorough breakdown of fats and complex molecules in your foods. This process is vital for preventing indigestion and ensuring that nutrients reach their necessary destinations; incorporating bitters into your diet can be transformative for anyone struggling with digestive sluggishness. Consider the common ***dandelion root***, often overlooked and uprooted as a garden nuisance. Yet, this humble plant is a powerhouse for digestion. Its bitter qualities stimulate digestive functions, making it an excellent remedy for those slow digestion days.

Creating your bitters can be rewarding, providing you with a personalized tool for digestive health. A simple recipe might include dandelion root, known for its liver-supportive properties, and gentian, one of the most potent herbal bitters. Start by macerating these herbs in a jar filled with a spirit such as vodka, which acts as a solvent, pulling out the active compounds from the herbs. Let this mixture sit in a cool, dark place for about a month, shaking it daily to promote extraction. After this period, strain the mixture, and your homemade bitters are ready. A few drops before meals can prime your digestive system and enhance overall digestive efficiency.

On the other hand, tonics nourish and support over more extended periods and are often used to maintain the health of the digestive system rather than treating acute problems. ***Turmeric*** is an excellent example of a tonic herb due to its anti-inflammatory properties. It can soothe chronic digestive inflammation and aid in gut health. Incorporating turmeric into your daily routine can be as simple as adding it to your meals. However, a turmeric tonic might be beneficial for a more directed approach. Mix turmeric powder with warm water, lemon juice, a pinch of black pepper (which enhances the absorption of curcumin in turmeric), and a teaspoon of honey to create a daily drink that supports your digestive system and overall inflammation levels.

Customizing bitters and tonics to suit your needs and taste preferences can elevate their effectiveness and make them more enjoyable.

If the intense bitterness of dandelion or gentian is overwhelming, consider blending them with milder-tasting herbs or natural sweeteners. Adding *ginger* or *cinnamon* can transform the flavour profile of your bitters, making them more palatable while retaining their digestive benefits. Similarly, for tonics, if turmeric's pungency is too much on its own, blending it with other supportive herbs like ginger or liquorice can improve the taste and enhance the anti-inflammatory and digestive benefits.

Incorporating these bitters and tonics into your daily routine does not have to be a chore. It can be as delightful and habitual as your morning coffee or tea. Over time, these bitters and tonics will not just support your digestion; they'll become a cornerstone of your wellness routine, gently nudging your body towards better health with every drop. As you explore and personalize your bitters and tonics, let them serve as a daily reminder of your commitment to nurturing your body with nature's gifts.

REMEDIES FOR ACID REFLUX AND HEARTBURN

When the discomfort of acid reflux strikes, it's as though your body is sending smoke signals from a fire within, reminding you of the delicate balance required to maintain digestive harmony. Among the soothing balm of herbal remedies, marshmallow root and slippery elm stand out for their demulcent properties, offering a protective layer to the irritated mucous membranes of your stomach and oesophagus. Imagine these herbs as gentle firefighters, using their soothing gel-like substances to coat the lining of your digestive tract, providing a barrier against the harsh acids that threaten its peace.

Marshmallow root, derived from the Althaea plant, produces a mucilage that acts almost like a soft gel when mixed with water. This mucilage coats and protects the tissues of the oesophagus and stomach, much like aloe vera soothes a sunburn. By forming this barrier, marshmallow root helps reduce the burning sensation often experienced with acid reflux. Similarly, *slippery elm*, which comes from the inner bark of the Ulmus rubra tree, creates a similar mucilage that coats the digestive tract. In addition to its soothing effect, it can stimulate nerve endings in the gastrointestinal tract to increase mucus secretion, which further helps protect the stomach lining from acidity.

On the other hand, *liquorice* operates through a slightly different mechanism, particularly in its deglycyrrhizinated form known as DGL, where glycyrrhizin (a sweet-tasting substance) has been removed. It soothes and coats the stomach lining and actively promotes the repair and regeneration of stomach and oesophagus tissues. DGL stimulates mucus production, creating a natural barrier against stomach acids. It's crucial, however, to choose DGL liquorice because it removes the compound glycyrrhizin, which can cause adverse effects like elevated blood pressure when taken in large quantities. Liquorice can be taken as a chewable tablet or as a tea, providing relief and aiding in the healing process of the affected mucous membranes.

Aloe vera, widely recognized for its cooling properties on the skin, plays a similar role in the digestive system. The gel from the aloe vera plant is rich in compounds that provide a soothing effect on the lining of the stomach and oesophagus. Drinking aloe vera juice can help calm the inflammation of gastroesophageal reflux disease (GERD) and speed up the healing process. The key is to look for pure, organic aloe vera juice free from aloin, which can be a laxative and irritate the digestive system.

While these herbal remedies offer significant relief, integrating lifestyle and dietary changes can enhance their effectiveness and prevent the recurrence of symptoms. Small, frequent meals can reduce the burden on your digestive system, preventing the overproduction of stomach acid. It's also beneficial to avoid lying down immediately after eating, as gravity keeps the stomach contents from moving upwards. Certain foods and beverages, such as caffeine, spicy, and alcohol, can trigger acid reflux. You should consume them in moderation or avoid them if they worsen your symptoms.

Incorporating gentle exercises into your routine can also improve digestion and reduce stress, often contributing to acid reflux. Techniques such as yoga or walking after meals can enhance gastric mobility and reduce stress levels, making it easier for your body to process food efficiently. Mindful eating habits such as eating slowly and chewing thoroughly make meals more enjoyable and aid in better digestion and nutrient absorption, which can help prevent heartburn discomfort.

By embracing these herbal remedies and lifestyle adjustments, you create a comprehensive approach to managing acid reflux and heartburn. This holistic strategy addresses the symptoms and contributes to a healthier digestive system, allowing you to enjoy your meals and life with less discomfort and more balance. As you continue to apply these practices, they become more than just treatments—they evolve into a lifestyle that honours your body's needs and fosters long-term digestive health.

COMBATING NAUSEA AND TRAVEL SICKNESS WITH HERBS

Navigating through the discomforts of nausea and travel sickness can often feel like an uphill battle, especially when you are on long journeys or facing morning sickness. Fortunately, nature offers us a bounty of remedies, with ginger and peppermint standing out for their remarkable ability to ease these upsets. Through their soothing properties, these herbs invite a sense of calm to the digestive system and help stabilize the inner sense of motion that can lead to nausea.

Various cultures have used *ginger* as a remedy for nausea and motion sickness for centuries due to its sharp, invigorating aroma and taste. Gingerol and shogaol are the main compounds that make ginger effective for reducing nausea. They promote the secretion of digestive enzymes that neutralize stomach acid and enhance gastrointestinal muscle movement. This helps to alleviate the feelings that lead to nausea. On the other hand, *peppermint* contains menthol, which is a natural analgesic and anti-inflammatory agent. This aids in relaxing the stomach muscles, reducing contractions that can lead to vomiting, and soothing the nerves associated with motion sickness.

Various preparation methods are available to integrate these herbs into your wellness routine, catering to different needs and preferences. Herbal teas are one of the simplest and most comforting ways to consume these herbs. A warm cup of ginger tea, perhaps with a touch of honey to soften the sharp taste, can be soothing before or during travel. With its refreshing flavour, peppermint tea is a cooling remedy, perfect for soothing an upset stomach on warm days or in warmer climates. For those who need quick, easy solutions, especially while travelling, capsules containing powdered ginger or peppermint oil provide a convenient alternative. They are easy to carry and can be taken with water whenever symptoms arise.

Incorporating these herbs as a preventative measure can significantly enhance their effectiveness. If you know you are prone to motion sickness or are expecting potential nausea, such as before a trip or during early pregnancy, taking a dose of ginger or peppermint about 30 minutes before you start travelling can help pre-empt the discomfort. Regular intake can build a more sustained resistance against nausea and motion sickness. For instance, starting your day with ginger tea might bolster your defences if you face a day that could trigger nausea.

Beyond the direct consumption of these herbs, additional supportive practices can enhance their effectiveness and provide further relief. *Acupressure*, for instance, derives from traditional

Chinese medicine and involves applying pressure to specific points on the body to reduce nausea symptoms. Notably, the P6 acupressure point on the inner forearm near the wrist effectively reduces nausea. Simple pressure applied with your fingers or an acupressure band can significantly relieve nausea or travel sickness.

Hydration also plays a crucial role in managing nausea, particularly during travel. Dehydration can exacerbate nausea symptoms, making them more challenging to control. Ensuring adequate fluid intake can help maintain your body's natural balance and enhance the effectiveness of herbal remedies. Infusing your water with slices of ginger or sprigs of peppermint can enhance the anti-nausea benefits while ensuring that you stay hydrated.

In this exploration of herbal remedies for combating nausea and travel sickness, ginger and peppermint's gentle yet powerful properties emerge as beacons of relief. Whether through teas, capsules, or the supportive practices of acupressure and adequate hydration, these herbs offer natural, practical solutions to help you navigate the discomforts of nausea and travel sickness, restoring your sense of well-being as you journey through life. With these tools, you are better equipped to face the challenges of motion-related discomforts, ensuring that your adventures and daily activities are marked more by joy and less by distress.

NATURAL PROBIOTICS: FERMENTED HERBS FOR GUT HEALTH

Exploring the realm of fermented herbs opens a delightful avenue to enhance gut health naturally. The fermentation process not only preserves the herbs but also amplifies their health benefits by infusing them with probiotics. These beneficial bacteria are crucial for maintaining a healthy digestive system, aiding digestion, and enhancing the immune system. Fermented herbal preparations can become a cornerstone of your wellness routine, offering a unique blend of flavours and health benefits that holistically support your digestive health.

Fermenting herbs at home is both an art and a science, accessible enough for beginners yet deep enough to offer a satisfying challenge to those more experienced in the culinary arts. To start, choose fresh and vibrant herbs, as their quality directly influences the quality of your final product. Herbs like **holy basil** and **lemon balm** are suitable for fermentation due to their robust flavours and inherent health properties. Holy basil, for instance, is known for its stress-reducing effects, while lemon balm can help soothe symptoms of indigestion.

To ferment these herbs:

1. Begin by washing them thoroughly to remove any dirt or impurities.
2. Chop the herbs coarsely to increase the surface area, aiding fermentation.
3. Place the chopped herbs in a clean jar, pressing them down lightly to compact them.
4. Prepare brine by dissolving sea salt in filtered water—approximately one tablespoon of salt per cup of water should suffice.
5. Pour the brine over the herbs until wholly submerged, leaving about an inch of space at the top of the jar. The herbs must stay submerged to prevent mould growth; you can use a fermentation weight or a smaller jar to keep them pressed down.
6. Cover the jar with a cloth or a fermentation lid to allow gases to escape. Let the jar sit at room temperature, away from direct sunlight, for about 2 to 3 weeks. During this time, the natural fermentation process will occur, with beneficial bacteria on the surface of the herbs multiplying

and converting sugars into lactic acid, preserving the
herbs and imbuing them with probiotics.

Incorporating these fermented herbs into your diet is an enjoyable way to boost your digestive health. The tangy flavour of fermented herbs makes them a delightful addition to meals, offering a unique taste that can enhance various dishes. Add fermented holy basil or lemon balm to salads, soups, or smoothies. You can also use the brine as a salad dressing or a marinade base, infusing your meals with probiotics and fermented herbs' deep, complex flavours.

As you become more accustomed to the flavours and benefits of fermented herbs, you may find yourself experimenting with different combinations and recipes. This exploratory process broadens your culinary repertoire and enhances your understanding of the health benefits of various herbs. Fermentation, a transformative process, mirrors the transformative effects these herbs can have on your health, particularly your digestive system.

In exploring fermented herbs for gut health, we've uncovered the profound benefits of incorporating these probiotic-rich preparations into your diet. From enhancing digestive health to boosting the immune system, fermented herbs offer a natural, flavourful way to support your body's wellness. As you integrate these practices into your daily routine, they become more than just dietary additions—they evolve into a foundational component of your holistic health strategy, emphasizing the power of natural processes and the efficacy of herbal remedies in maintaining health and vitality.

As we conclude this chapter on herbal remedies for digestive health, we've journeyed through the soothing realms of teas, explored natural solutions for common digestive issues, delved into the potent world of bitters and tonics, and discovered specific herbs' protective and healing properties.

Each section has equipped you with knowledge and practical solutions to enhance your digestive wellness naturally and effectively. In the next chapter, we will transition from the digestive system to exploring herbal remedies that boost immunity, a timely and critical aspect of maintaining health in a world where well-being is increasingly cherished.

CHAPTER 5

Boosting Immunity with Herbs

I n the tapestry of health, our immune system acts like a vigilant gardener, tending to our body's needs and protecting it from harmful invaders. Imagine this system as an intricate network of pathways lined with defenders poised to counter threats and maintain balance. Yet, even the most diligent gardeners need support to replenish their resources and strengthen their defences. This is where the power of herbs comes into play, offering natural reinforcements that enhance our body's ability to protect itself. In this chapter, we explore some of nature's most potent antiviral herbs that serve as allies in our quest for robust health, weaving their protective qualities into the fabric of our daily lives to fortify our immune defences.

ANTIVIRAL HERBS AND HOW TO USE THEM

Elderberry's Antiviral Effects

Elderberry, a small, dark berry from the Sambucus tree, is rich in flavour and packed with antiviral properties, making it a formidable foe against colds and flu. The magic of elderberry lies in its bioflavonoids and other proteins that effectively disarm viruses, stopping them from invading healthy cells. This berry is particularly adept at tackling the influenza virus, shortening its unwelcome stay in our bodies. Elderberry contains compounds like flavonoids, particularly anthocyanins that can block the virus's ability to enter and infect host cells. These compounds interfere with the virus's attachment to the cell surface, preventing it from penetrating the cell membrane. When you feel the onset of flu symptoms, a syrup made from these potent berries can be your first line of defence, reducing the severity and duration of the illness.

To harness the full potential of elderberry, consider preparing a simple homemade syrup. Begin by simmering dried elderberries with water, a slice of ginger, and some cloves—this extracts the active components and adds an extra layer of immune support with the antiseptic properties of ginger and cloves. After approximately 45 minutes, strain the mixture and incorporate honey for its soothing and antibacterial properties. You can store this syrup in your refrigerator and take it daily during flu season to boost your immune system or consume it every few hours at the first sign of illness.

Echinacea's Immune Support

Echinacea, often pictured in the vibrant hues of purple coneflower, is widely respected for its immune-boosting capabilities. It works by increasing the production of white blood cells, which play a critical role in fighting infections. Moreover, echinacea increases the output of interferon, a vital part of the body's response to viral infections. Its benefits are best realized at the onset of cold or flu symptoms, acting as a catalyst for the body's natural defence mechanisms.

For practical use, you can take echinacea as a tincture or tea. Due to its concentration, a tincture might provide a more potent dose, which can be crucial at the first sign of illness. If you prefer a milder approach, brewing tea from dried echinacea flowers can also support your immune system. Take echinacea at the first signs of illness and continue for 7 to 10 days to help boost your immune system's response.

Andrographis for Respiratory Health

Andrographis, known as the "King of Bitters," is an herb cherished in traditional Chinese and Ayurvedic medicine for its strong antiviral and antibacterial properties. It is particularly effective in treating respiratory infections, where it helps reduce inflammation, clear congestion, and boost the immune response. Given its potency, Andrographis is an excellent herb to include during respiratory virus season or at the first hint of respiratory discomfort.

A standard approach to incorporating Andrographis into your immune defence strategy is through capsules or tablets, which are commonly available and provide a controlled dose of the herb. Due to its bitter flavour, this may be preferable to a tincture or tea for most people.

Preparation and Dosage Guidelines

When preparing and using antiviral herbs, it's essential to follow specific guidelines to ensure their efficacy and safety. Dosages can vary based on the form of the herb (dried, tincture, capsule) and the specifics of the individual taking them, including age, health status, and the presence of any underlying conditions. Always start with the lowest possible dose to see how your body responds, and consult with a healthcare provider, especially if you are pregnant, nursing, or on medication.

For elderberry syrup, a general recommendation is 1-2 tablespoons per day for immune support during cold and flu season and the same amount every 4 hours at the onset of flu symptoms. For echinacea and Andrographis, follow the product label's dosing instructions or consult a professional herbalist to determine the appropriate amount based on your specific health needs.

Incorporating these antiviral herbs into your daily routine during peak viral seasons or at the initial signs of viral symptoms can significantly bolster your immune defences. By understanding the properties of each herb and adhering to recommended preparations and dosages, you empower yourself to navigate the challenges of cold and flu season with natural and practical solutions at your fingertips. Integrating these herbs into your life becomes more than mere supplements—they are part of a holistic wellness approach that honours the body's natural rhythms and healing capabilities.

HERBAL STRATEGIES FOR COLD AND FLU SEASON

When the chill of the cold and flu season begins to whisper through our homes and communities, it's not just the drop in temperature we must prepare for but the rise in common colds and flu cases that often accompany it. Nurturing your immune system during this time becomes not just a practice but a priority. Herbal teas, with their soothing warmth and medicinal properties, are a cornerstone of preventive health strategies during these vulnerable months. One such tea, which I often recommend, combines the immune-boosting power of liquorice root, marshmallow root's soothing properties, and cinnamon's warmth. ***Liquorice root*** is a potent antiviral and antimicrobial agent; marshmallow root coats and soothes the throat and gut. ***Cinnamon*** adds a warming touch that helps to improve circulation, which is vital for immune function. To prepare this tea, simmer a teaspoon of each dried liquorice, ***marshmallow root***, and cinnamon stick in two cups of water for about 15 minutes. Strain the mixture and enjoy it warm, perhaps with a dollop of raw honey, adding antibacterial properties to this strengthening drink. This tea can be consumed daily during the cold season to help fortify the body against viral infections.

Moreover, herbal steam inhalation introduces another layer of defence, particularly effective in clearing nasal passages and easing respiratory discomfort. **Thyme** and **eucalyptus**, for example, are rich in essential oils that are particularly effective at thinning mucus and providing antibacterial benefits. To create a therapeutic steam inhalation:

1. Bring a large pot of water to a simmer. Add a handful of thyme leaves and a few drops of eucalyptus oil.
2. Remove the pot from the heat, lean over it, and drape a towel over your head to trap the steam.
3. Inhale deeply for about 10 minutes. This practice can be particularly soothing before bed, helping clear the passages and making sleep more restful and healing.

In the realm of tinctures, the combination of astragalus and reishi mushroom creates a powerful ally for immune support. Both herbs are known for their immune-modulating solid effects. They can accommodate building resilience over the colder months. To prepare a tincture:

1. Fill a jar one-third full with dried astragalus root and reishi mushroom slices.
2. Cover the herbs entirely with a neutral spirit like vodka, ensuring there are about two inches of alcohol above the level of the herbs.
3. Seal the jar and allow it to sit in a cool, dark place for about six to eight weeks, shaking it daily.
4. After the maceration period, strain the tincture through a cheesecloth into dark glass dropper bottles.
5. For immune support, take 30-40 drops of this tincture in a bit of water once daily throughout the flu season.

Lastly, topical applications of herbal remedies can provide symptomatic relief during bouts of cold and flu. Eucalyptus chest rubs, for instance, offer a comforting and effective method for easing respiratory discomfort. To make a simple eucalyptus chest rub, start with a base of about two tablespoons of coconut oil, warmed slightly to soften. Add ten drops of eucalyptus essential oil and five drops of peppermint essential oil. Both oils are known for their decongestant properties and ability to soothe coughs and open respiratory pathways. Mix well and apply a small amount to the chest and back as needed, especially before sleep, to aid a restful night with easier breathing.

These herbal strategies provide a comforting, natural way to enhance your immune defences during the cold and flu season. Whether through the daily ritual of sipping a warm herbal tea, the soothing practice of steam inhalation, the resilience-building properties of tincture intake, or the direct relief offered by topical applications, these practices weave together a tapestry of preventive care that supports your body's natural defences, keeping you and your loved ones more resilient through the winter months.

ADAPTOGENS: NATURE'S STRESS RELIEVERS AND IMMUNE BOOSTERS

In the lush, verdant corners of the world, where nature thrives in its wildest forms, grow some of the most remarkable plants known to human health—adaptogens. These botanicals uniquely enhance your body's resistance to stress while balancing your biological functions. The term "adaptogen" was coined to describe herbs that increase the body's ability to adapt to environmental and psychological stresses, thus promoting better overall health and well-being. They act at a molecular level by moderating the hypothalamic-pituitary-adrenal (HPA) axis and the sympathoadrenal system, which are involved in the body's response to stress. This modulation helps enhance your immune function, as stress directly impacts your immune response. The beauty of adaptogens lies in their dual action: they calm you when you're stressed and boost your energy when you're fatigued, always working toward optimal homeostasis.

Ashwagandha, a revered herb in the Ayurvedic tradition, exemplifies the power of adaptogens. Known scientifically as *Withania somnifera*, it provides a sterling example of how adaptogens support resilience and stamina. Ashwagandha increases energy levels and alleviates stress. It achieves this by stabilising blood sugar and reducing cortisol levels, often elevated during stressful periods. Incorporating ashwagandha into your routine can be transformative for those facing daily pressures, whether from work, family, or health challenges. It supports physical endurance and recovery from fatigue. It promotes mental clarity and focus, making it a cornerstone herb for anyone looking to sustain high-performance levels in all areas of life.

Holy basil, or Tulsi, affectionately known in India, is another stellar adaptogen that brings profound benefits, particularly in reducing stress and enhancing cognitive function. This herb is a nerve tonic with a slight stimulant effect that can elevate your mood and spirit. It's beneficial for those who find themselves mentally overwhelmed. Holy basil helps protect organs and tissues against chemical stress from pollutants and heavy metals, which are part of modern life's unavoidable burdens. Furthermore, its anti-inflammatory effects can soothe the nerves, reducing the feelings of anxiety and stress that often cloud mental clarity.

Incorporating adaptogens like rhodiola and Schisandra into your daily health routines can help you maintain balance and vitality. *Rhodiola rosea*, often found in the cold mountainous regions of Europe and Asia, is renowned for enhancing physical and mental stamina. It sharpens focus under stress and can reduce fatigue significantly. Starting your day with a rhodiola supplement can invigorate your morning routine, providing the stamina needed to tackle a demanding day. ***Schisandra***, a berry used for centuries in Traditional Chinese Medicine, supports adrenal function, which is crucial in responding to stress. It also protects the liver, promoting the efficient clearance of toxins that can accumulate during stressful times. Integrating Schisandra into your regimen can be as simple as taking a few dried berries each day or brewing them into a tea, offering a straightforward method to bolster your resilience against daily stresses.

By weaving these adaptogens into the fabric of your daily life, you proactively approach health beyond mere reaction to symptoms. Adaptogens provide a foundation of resilience that supports your body's ability to thrive in the face of life's inevitable stresses. They are not just remedies but potent allies that enhance your body's innate capacities, promoting a life of balance, health, and sustained vitality. As you continue exploring these plants' profound benefits, let their natural strengths remind you of your resilience and adaptability.

NUTRITIVE HERBS TO SUPPORT OVERALL IMMUNITY

In the lush landscape of herbal medicine, certain plants are treasured not just for their ability to heal but for their profound capacity to nourish and fortify the body. Among these, nettle stands out with its decadent array of vitamins and minerals, making it an excellent ally for immune health. It is often overlooked due to its stinging reputation when fresh nettle, processed into teas or supplements, unfolds as a nutritional powerhouse. Rich in vitamins A, C, and K and several B vitamins and minerals like iron, calcium, magnesium, and potassium, nettle provides a broad spectrum of nutrients essential for maintaining a robust immune system. Its high iron content prevents anaemia, a common issue that can impair immune function. To incorporate nettle into your daily routine, consider a simple nettle tea. Just steep dried nettle leaves in boiling water for about 10 minutes and enjoy a mineral-rich infusion that nourishes your body intensely, supporting immune function and overall vitality.

Astragalus root, with its sweet, earthy flavour, offers another layer of deep immune support. Used for centuries in Traditional Chinese Medicine, Astragalus works by increasing the body's production of white blood cells, which are crucial in fighting pathogens. Additionally, it enhances the body's interferon production, a key player in the immune response to viral infections. Astragalus is particularly valuable for building and maintaining a resilient immune system over the long term. Integrating Astragalus into your diet can be as simple as adding the dried root to soups, which lends a mild, pleasant flavour, or taking it as a supplement when you feel particularly vulnerable to illness.

Sea buckthorn, a vibrant berry known for its high antioxidant content, is another jewel in the crown of immune-supporting herbs. Antioxidants protect the body from oxidative stress and inflammation, which can weaken the immune system. Sea buckthorn contains vitamins C and E, powerful antioxidants and other nutrients supporting immune health. Its omega-7 fatty acids, rare in the plant kingdom, also promote healthy skin, which serves as a critical first line of defence against environmental pathogens. For a quick boost, a spoonful of sea buckthorn berry oil can be taken each day as a dietary supplement, providing a concentrated dose of its protective nutrients.

Creating a Nutritive Herbal Infusion

To harness the combined benefits of these and other nutritional herbs, consider preparing a nourishing herbal infusion that serves as a daily tonic to fortify your immune system. Start with equal parts of dried nettle, oat straw, and red clover, each herb bringing its unique blend of vitamins and minerals to the mix. Oatstraw, rich in magnesium and silica, supports nerve health and resilience to stress. At the same time, red clover, with its isoflavones and phytosterols, enhances hormonal balance and offers additional immune support.

To prepare the infusion:

1. Add a quarter cup of the mixed dried herbs to a quart of boiling water.
2. Let this steep overnight, or at least four hours, to extract the full spectrum of water-soluble nutrients.
3. Strain the mixture in the morning, squeezing the herbs to extract every drop of the nutrient-dense liquid. You can enjoy this infusion throughout the day, perhaps with a splash of lemon for added flavour and vitamin C, ensuring your body receives a continuous supply of immune-supporting nutrients.

By incorporating these nutritive herbs into your daily wellness routine, you actively build a foundation of health that prepares your body to fend off transient illnesses and supports robust, long-term immune function. This holistic approach to health, emphasising prevention and nourishment, mirrors the broader principles of herbal medicine, which advocate for harmony and balance in all aspects of life.

In concluding this chapter on boosting immunity with herbs, we have looked at various strategies. These include using potent antivirals and adaptogens and integrating deeply nourishing herbs that strengthen your immune system. As you go through the ideas in this chapter, let them encourage you to take a proactive approach to wellness that emphasises nurturing vitality and resilience rather than solely fighting illness. The next chapter will delve into the soothing and therapeutic realm of herbal remedies for skin and beauty. This will expand our focus from internal health to external healing and care, furthering our journey towards holistic wellness.

"When we give others the knowledge of herbs, we empower them to take charge of their own health." - Juliette de Bairacli Levy

People who give without expecting anything in return live happier lives. So, let's make a difference together!

Would you help someone just like you—curious about herbal remedies and natural medicine but unsure where to start?

My mission is to make herbal remedies and natural medicine easy and fun for everyone. But to reach more people, I need your help.

Most people choose books based on reviews. So, I'm asking you to help a fellow herbalist by leaving a review.

It costs nothing and takes less than a minute, but it could change someone's journey with herbal remedies and natural medicine. Your review could help...

- ...inspire healthy living
- ...promote environmentally friendly practices
- ...others discover a natural way to boost their health.
- ...transform someone's life.

To make a difference, simply scan the QR code below and leave a review:

If you love helping others, you're my kind of person.
Thank you from the bottom of my heart!
Thank you for taking the time to share your thoughts.
Your generosity can truly make a difference!

Sage Wilder

CHAPTER 6

Skin and Beauty – Natural Care

As we gently unfold the petals of herbal wisdom in our exploration of natural health, we arrive at a sanctuary where beauty and wellness converge—our skin. The skin, a vast and tender landscape, mirrors our internal health and external interactions. It breathes, protects, and reveals, responding to life's rhythms and exposures. In this chapter, I invite you into a nurturing space where we harness the gentle power of herbal infusions to rejuvenate, heal, and protect your skin, transforming everyday skincare into a ritual of deep self-care and connection with nature.

HERBAL INFUSIONS FOR RADIANT SKIN

Calendula for Skin Repair

Imagine a golden bloom under the sun: its petals are vibrant with life and energy. This is calendula, a marigold with an essence that is healing and bright in appearance. **Calendula** is cherished in herbal skincare for its noteworthy healing properties. When infused in water or oil, calendula flowers release anti-inflammatory compounds that soothe the skin, reduce redness, and promote rapid healing of cuts, wounds, and irritations. Its ability to enhance collagen production makes it invaluable in repairing the skin, not just on the surface but also deep within, where true healing begins.

For those navigating the complexities of skin conditions such as eczema or psoriasis, calendula offers relief. Its gentle, soothing effect can calm inflamed tissues and support the skin's natural healing process. Consider preparing a simple calendula infusion to incorporate the healing power into your skincare routine. Steep dried calendula petals in hot water for about 15 minutes, strain, and let it cool. This golden infusion can be used as a facial rinse in the morning to awaken and soothe your skin or as a compress on irritated areas to harness its healing properties.

Chamomile's Soothing Properties

Chamomile, with its delicate blossoms and sweet, earthy aroma, is a tea for calming the mind and a balm for soothing the skin. Chamomile infusions are known for their anti-inflammatory and antioxidant properties, which can help alleviate skin irritations and protect against environmental damage. Its gentle nature makes it suitable for even the most sensitive skin, reducing redness and providing a soothing effect that can help ease the stresses of your day as it touches your skin.

For those evenings when you feel the day's wear weigh heavily on your skin, a chamomile infusion can be your release ritual. Brew a strong infusion of chamomile flowers, let it cool, then soak a soft cloth or cotton pad in this soothing elixir. Apply it to your face as a calming compress, allowing the sweet aroma and cooling touch to melt away tension and inflammation. It's a simple yet profoundly nurturing way to end your day, reconnecting with yourself and nature.

. . .

Green Tea for Antioxidant Protection

Green tea, revered for its health benefits when sipped, also offers a potent shield for your skin when applied topically. Rich in polyphenols, green tea is a powerful antioxidant that protects the skin from free radicals and sun damage. Incorporating green tea into your skincare helps delay signs of ageing and improves skin tone and elasticity.

Imagine starting your day with the protective power of green tea. Prepare a green tea infusion by steeping tea leaves in hot water (not boiling), then let it cool. Use this infusion as a morning facial rinse to harness its antioxidant power, which can protect and refresh your skin throughout the day. For an added boost, freeze the infusion in ice cube trays and use a green tea ice cube as a refreshing facial rub in the morning. This invigorates the skin and enhances circulation, giving you a natural glow that speaks of vitality and care.

Infusion Recipes for Different Skin Types

Every skin type has its own unique needs and stories. Whether dry, oily, or sensitive skin, herbal infusions can be customized to meet your requirements. For example, a blend of calendula and marshmallow root can provide deep hydration and healing for dry skin. Steep these herbs together, strain and use the infusion as a base for a hydrating face mask or a daily moisturizer. Oily skin, on the other hand, may benefit from an infusion of green tea and **witch hazel**, which can help regulate oil production and tighten pores. For sensitive skin, a soothing blend of **chamomile** and **lavender** can calm irritations and reduce redness. Mix these herbs, steep, strain, and use the infusion as a gentle facial wash or toner.

As you integrate these herbal infusions into your skincare rituals, let each application be a moment of connection with the healing power of plants. Let it be a time when you nourish your skin and honour the natural beauty that flows within you.

NATURAL REMEDIES FOR ACNE AND ECZEMA

Navigating the often turbulent waters of skin conditions such as acne and eczema can feel daunting. However, nature provides potent remedies that alleviate these conditions and nurture the skin, enhancing its natural balance and beauty. Tea tree oil and neem stand out as powerful allies in the fight against acne. At the same time, soothing herbal baths offer a gentle solution for the discomfort of eczema. Furthermore, understanding and adjusting your diet can play a crucial role in managing these skin conditions, highlighting the integral connection between what we consume and the health of our skin.

Tea Tree Oil's Antimicrobial Action

Tea tree oil, obtained through the distillation of the leaves of the Melaleuca alternifolia tree, a species native to Australia, has been valued for its potent antimicrobial and anti-inflammatory properties for generations by indigenous communities. When it comes to acne, tea tree oil performs admirably, acting as a natural antiseptic that effectively combats acne-causing bacteria. Its ability to penetrate and disinfect the pores makes it an invaluable tool for clearing skin.

To incorporate tea tree oil into your acne care routine:

1. Consider a simple, homemade spot treatment.
2. Mix a few drops of tea tree oil with a teaspoon of witch hazel. This gentle carrier enhances the oil's antibacterial actions.
3. Apply this mixture directly to pimples using a clean cotton swab.

This targeted approach helps to reduce inflammation and clear up blemishes without the harshness of commercial acne treatments, which can strip the skin of its natural oils and exacerbate the problem. However, it's important to note that tea tree oil is potent and should always be diluted to prevent skin irritation. Patch testing on a small skin area before application is recommended to ensure compatibility.

Neem for Skin Clarity

Neem is an evergreen tree originating from the Indian subcontinent. It provides numerous advantages for skin health, especially for individuals struggling with acne. The neem leaf, rich in antibacterial and anti-inflammatory properties, is an excellent natural remedy for acne. Its components effectively target and reduce acne-causing bacteria and inflammation, promoting more transparent, healthier skin. Moreover, neem helps regulate oil production, which can significantly affect acne outbreaks.

Creating a neem face mask can be an effective way to harness its benefits for acne-prone skin. To prepare, make a paste by grinding dried neem leaves with water or mixing neem powder with yoghurt to create a soothing face mask. Apply the mask to clean, dry skin, leave it on for about 15 minutes, then rinse with warm water. This treatment can help purify the skin, reduce breakouts, and restore a natural, healthy glow.

Herbal Baths for Eczema Relief

For those experiencing the often intense discomfort of eczema, herbal baths can offer much-needed relief. Herbs like oats and lavender are particularly beneficial, providing soothing, anti-inflammatory, and healing properties. For centuries, people have turned to *oatmeal* to soothe irritated skin and alleviate itching, making it an ideal solution for managing eczema flare-ups. *Lavender*, renowned for its soothing scent and anti-inflammatory effects, can help reduce redness and irritation.

To prepare a therapeutic herbal bath:

1. Start by grinding a cup of plain oats in a blender until you have a fine powder.
2. Add this to a warm bath along with a handful of dried lavender flowers.
3. Soak in this gentle bath for about 15 to 20 minutes, allowing the properties of the oats and lavender to soothe your skin.
4. Pat your skin dry gently and follow up with a natural moisturizer to lock in hydration. This natural treatment can significantly reduce the itchiness and discomfort associated with eczema, making it a gentle alternative to more aggressive treatments.

In addition, Dead Sea Salts provide great relief for Eczema sufferers and are one of my favourite bath ingredients, especially on flare-up days.

Dietary Considerations for Skin Health

The adage "you are what you eat" holds profound truth regarding skin health. Your diet directly affects your skin's appearance and ability to fight conditions like acne and eczema. Incorporating foods rich in **omega-3** fatty acids, such as salmon, flaxseeds, and walnuts, can help reduce inflammation in the body, including the skin. Additionally, ensuring a plentiful intake of fruits and vegetables, which are high in antioxidants and vitamins, can support skin healing and reduce oxidative stress that might exacerbate skin issues.

Supplementing your diet with herbs like **turmeric** and **ginger** can also offer benefits due to their anti-inflammatory properties. Consider incorporating a daily turmeric latte or adding fresh ginger to your meals to enhance your dietary approach to skin health. Remember, a balanced diet that supports your skin's needs can be a fundamental step in managing skin conditions and improving overall skin health.

When dealing with allergy-induced skin irritations, it's crucial to take a systematic approach. Keeping a detailed food diary to track what you eat and monitoring your skin condition can provide valuable insights into your allergies. Discussing your symptoms and findings with a specialist who can offer expert guidance is also essential. For example, over time, I've become aware of my sensitivity to dairy, particularly cheese; I noticed that after consuming dairy, I would develop a rash a few hours later. I switched to drinking oat milk to address this issue, which has helped me avoid these reactions.

As we explore these natural remedies and dietary adjustments, remember that each step you take moves towards clearer and healthier skin and a more profound harmony within your body. These methods, steeped in nature's wisdom, offer more than symptom relief; they invite you into a balanced way of living where your external beauty and internal health are naturally intertwined.

ANTI-AGING HERBS AND RECIPES FOR SKIN CARE

In the lush gardens of herbal care, where each plant offers a snippet of age-old wisdom, lie secrets to maintaining youthful vibrancy and skin elasticity. As we gracefully adapt to the natural ageing process, it becomes essential to seek allies in nature that slow the external signs of ageing and nurture our skin deeply, enhancing its innate ability to renew and recover. Among these allies, gotu kola and ginkgo biloba stand out for their rich antioxidant profiles, playing pivotal roles in skin care regimens focused on longevity and health.

Gotu kola, a staple in Ayurvedic and traditional Chinese medicine, is celebrated for its therapeutic benefits and potent anti-ageing properties. This herb helps stimulate collagen production, which is crucial for maintaining skin elasticity and strength. As collagen naturally depletes with age, gotu kola's ability to boost its synthesis is invaluable. Moreover, it enhances the formation of new skin cells, aiding in the repair and maintenance of healthy skin. Consider a simple homemade serum for those looking to integrate the benefits of gotu kola into your daily routine. Start by infusing dried gotu kola leaves in a carrier oil like jojoba or almond for a few weeks, allowing the oil to absorb the herb's properties. Strain the mixture and apply a few drops of this enriched oil to your face before bedtime, massaging gently. This nightly ritual provides your skin with essential nutrients and improves blood circulation, enhancing overall skin health and appearance.

Ginkgo biloba, another venerable herb, offers a treasure trove of flavonoids and terpenoids, antioxidants known for their practical free radical-scavenging abilities. Environmental stressors such as pollution and UV radiation can accelerate skin ageing by generating free radicals. Ginkgo's antioxidant properties help protect the skin from these stressors, reducing premature ageing and maintaining skin vitality. A refreshing ginkgo facial mist can be a delightful way to incorporate this herb into your skincare. Brew a strong infusion of ginkgo biloba leaves, let it cool, then pour it into a clean spray bottle, perhaps with a splash of rosewater for its soothing properties. Use this mist throughout the day to refresh your skin and provide a continuous shield against environmental damage.

Shifting the focus from prevention to rejuvenation, ***rosehip oil*** has become a highly regenerative natural oil for mature skin. This oil is extracted from the seeds of wild rose bushes and is rich in vitamins A and C, both known for their roles in skin cell regeneration. Vitamin A, or retinol, encourages skin cell turnover. In contrast, vitamin C enhances collagen production, which is vital for reducing the appearance of wrinkles and fine lines. Applying rosehip oil can dramatically improve skin texture and tone, giving it a youthful appearance. Apply a few drops of pure rosehip oil to your face at night, gently massaging it into the skin. The oil moisturizes and works overnight to repair and rejuvenate skin cells, helping you wake up with a revitalized complexion. As with any oil, if using Rosehip for the first time, it is advisable to perform a patch test. To do this, apply a small amount of the oil to a small section of your skin, i.e., the palm side of your wrist, then wait 24 hours for any reaction.

Preparing homemade anti-ageing masks can be fun and effective for those who love crafting skincare solutions. These masks can be tailored to your skin's needs, incorporating various anti-ageing herbs and natural ingredients. For a hydrating and firming mask, blend cooked oatmeal with honey and a strong infusion of green tea. Oatmeal soothes and hydrates the skin, honey provides natural antibacterial properties, and green tea offers antioxidant protection. Apply this mask to your face once a week for deep nourishment and protection.

Beyond topical applications, embracing a lifestyle that promotes healthy ageing is equally essential. Regular hydration, adequate sleep, stress management, and a diet rich in fruits, vegetables, and healthy fats contribute to skin health. Regular physical activity can improve circulation, bringing more oxygen and nutrients to your skin. Mindfulness practices like yoga or meditation can help manage stress, which often manifests in our skin's health. Integrating these lifestyle habits with your herbal skincare regimen creates a holistic approach to beauty that radiates from the inside out.

NATURAL HERBS FOR HEALTHY HAIR GROWTH AND SHINE

Stimulating Hair Growth with Rosemary and Peppermint

In the lush garden of herbal remedies that cater to skin health, let's not overlook those that lavish similar benefits upon our hair. ***Rosemary***, for instance, is a culinary delight and a potent tonic for stimulating hair growth and enhancing scalp health. Its primary mechanism is improving blood circulation to the scalp, which fosters hair follicle activity and promotes stronger, healthier hair growth. ***Peppermint***, similarly, invigorates the scalp with its tingling essence, awakening dormant hair follicles and encouraging growth. This is due to its high content of menthol, which increases blood flow to the area it's applied to.

Consider making a stimulating scalp massage oil to incorporate:

1. Consider these herbs in your hair care regimen (Rosemary and Peppermint).
2. Start by infusing carrier oil, such as coconut or jojoba, with dried rosemary and peppermint leaves.
3. Let this mixture sit in a warm, dark place for a week or two, allowing the oils to draw out the active ingredients from the herbs.
4. Once your infusion is ready, massage it gently into your scalp a few nights a week.

Not only does this stimulate blood flow, but it also nourishes the roots with herbal benefits, setting the stage for vibrant hair growth.

Horsetail for Hair Strength

When we consider hair's structural integrity, horsetail is an outstanding herb. This ancient plant is rich in silica, a mineral known for strengthening hair, improving its texture, and reducing brittleness. This mineral helps to fortify the hair strands from within, ensuring that each shaft is robust and less prone to breakage. Horsetail's benefits extend to improving the sheen and vitality of your hair, giving it a healthy, glossy appearance that radiates with natural health.

Incorporating horsetail into your hair care routine can be as straightforward as preparing a horsetail hair rinse. Simmer dried horsetail in water for about 20 minutes, strain the liquid, and allow it to cool. After shampooing, use this herbal rinse to treat your hair. Its mineral-rich properties strengthen the hair and enhance its natural lustre. Regular use can significantly change the quality and texture of your hair, reflecting the deep nourishment it provides.

Aloe Vera for Moisture and Conditioning

Aloe vera is well-known for its soothing properties on the skin, but its benefits for hair are equally impressive. It is renowned for its hydrating properties, particularly beneficial for individuals with dry and damaged hair. It deeply moisturizes the hair shaft, providing hydration from the roots to the tips. Furthermore, aloe vera helps to smooth the hair cuticle, enhancing shine and reducing frizz, making it an excellent conditioner.

For an easy home remedy, apply the gel from an aloe vera leaf directly to your hair and scalp. Leave it on as a mask for about 30 minutes before rinsing. This treatment deeply conditions your hair and soothes the scalp, reducing dandruff and irritation. Aloe vera's gentle, nourishing properties make it suitable for all hair types, ensuring everyone can embrace its hydrating benefits.

Natural Dyes and Highlights from Herbs

When it comes to hair care and colour, it's important to consider natural alternatives that are gentle and healthy. **Chamomile** and **henna** are beautiful herbs that provide a kind and nurturing option for those seeking to avoid harsh chemical dyes. Chamomile can enhance the golden tones of lighter hair, giving strands a sun-kissed glow. Prepare a strong infusion of chamomile flowers, let it cool, then use it as a final rinse after shampooing to enhance your natural highlights gradually. For those desiring richer, darker tones, henna provides a deep, vibrant colour while conditioning the hair. Mix into a paste with some lemon juice and apply to the hair; henna dyes and strengthens each strand.

Herbal Rinses and Oils for Nourishing the Scalp

Lastly, herbal rinses and oils can transform your hair care routine into a nourishing ritual. Infuse herbs such as **lavender** and **rosemary** into your hair rinses to help balance scalp oil production and promote healthier, more luscious hair. These rinses used post-shampoo, impart aromatic and therapeutic qualities to your hair care routine, turning it into a moment of relaxation and self-care.

Preventing Hair Loss Through Herbal Remedies

In addressing hair loss, herbs like saw **palmetto** and **nettle root** come into play, offering natural remedies to help prevent this common issue. These herbs block the production of DHT, a hormone associated with hair loss. Integrating these herbs through teas or supplements can provide internal support against hair thinning.

Nutritional Support for Hair Health

Supporting hair health extends beyond topical treatments to include nutritional support. Incorporating herbs like **ginseng** and **flaxseeds**, rich in nutrients that stimulate hair growth and health, can make a significant difference. Drinking ginseng tea or adding ground flaxseeds to your meals can give your hair the nutrition it needs to thrive.

In nurturing your hair with these herbal remedies and practices, you embrace a holistic approach to beauty that enhances your appearance and cares deeply for your natural well-being. This chapter invites you to weave these herbal treasures into your daily life, improving the health and beauty of your hair naturally and joyfully.

In this chapter, we have covered natural hair and skin care and seen how herbs can improve the health and look of our skin and hair and overall well-being. By opting for natural remedies, we are embracing a sustainable and health-focused approach to beauty. In the next chapter, we will discuss strategies for coping with stress and anxiety as part of our ongoing journey towards holistic wellness.

CHAPTER 7

Mental Health and Wellbeing

As we navigate the ebb and flow of daily life, our mental and emotional well-being often takes a backseat. We manage deadlines, family duties, and personal challenges while maintaining a semblance of balance. Yet, the stress and anxiety induced by our bustling lives can accumulate beneath the surface, silently impacting our health. In this chapter, we focus on the gentle power of herbal remedies. This natural arsenal can support, soothe, and stabilize our mental and emotional landscapes.

HERBS FOR ANXIETY AND STRESS RELIEF

Lavender for Relaxation

Imagine a field of lavender, its vibrant hues under the sun, the air aromatic with its calming scent. This image alone might soothe your senses, but the true magic of lavender lies in its profound ability to calm the mind and alleviate stress. Lavender, scientifically known as *Lavandula angustifolia*, has been revered through the ages not just for its delightful fragrance but also for its medicinal properties, particularly its anxiolytic (anxiety-reducing) effects. Whether used in teas, in essential oil form, or as a part of aromatherapy practices, lavender acts as a nervous system relaxant, easing anxiety and promoting a sense of well-being.

To integrate lavender into your stress management routine, consider keeping a vial of essential oil at your desk or bedside. A simple inhalation of its scent can serve as a quick reset to a stressful moment, gently coaxing your nervous system back to calm. Alternatively, brewing lavender tea in the evening can help unwind your thoughts and prepare you for a restful night.

Lemon Balm's Mood-Enhancing Properties

Next, let's explore the cheerful world of lemon balm or *Melissa officinalis*. With its lemony scent and flavour, this herb has been used since the Middle Ages to improve mood and cognitive function. The leaves contain compounds with a mild sedative effect, making lemon balm an excellent choice for those who experience anxiety or stressful moods. Its ability to enhance the mood while simultaneously reducing anxiety creates a favourable environment for mental clarity and calmness.

For those moments when you feel overwhelmed or moody, a cup of lemon balm tea can be a soothing balm. Its preparation is simple: steep fresh or dried lemon balm leaves in boiling water for 10 minutes, strain, and enjoy. This herbal tea not only lifts your spirits but also gently soothes your nerves, allowing you to navigate your day with a lighter heart and a clearer mind.

Passionflower for Better Sleep

Transitioning to the world of sleep, Passionflower, or *Passiflora incarnata*, emerges as a key player. Known for its beautiful flowers, Passionflower has been traditionally used to treat anxiety and insomnia. Its calming effects on the central nervous system make it an effective herb for improving sleep quality and reducing nighttime awakenings, addressing a common symptom of anxiety—disrupted sleep.

Incorporating Passionflower into your nighttime routine can help you disconnect from the day's stresses and ease into a peaceful sleep. You can take Passionflower as a tea or in extract form. For tea, steep dried Passionflower in hot water for about 15 minutes before bedtime. If you prefer a more potent remedy, take passionflower extract in drops or capsules according to the product label's dosage instructions.

Guidelines for Using Anxiolytic Herbs

While these herbs have robust benefits, it's crucial to approach their use with mindfulness, especially regarding dosing and potential interactions with other medications. Always start with the lowest possible dose to see how your body responds. If you are currently taking medication for anxiety or any other condition, consult with your healthcare provider before incorporating these herbs into your regimen. This ensures that the herbs complement rather than complicate your existing treatment plan.

Moreover, while herbs can significantly aid in managing stress and anxiety, they are most effective when used as part of a broader approach to mental health that includes healthy lifestyle choices such as regular physical activity, a balanced diet, and adequate sleep. Herbs are not a cure-all but a supportive component in the holistic care of your mental well-being.

In this chapter, as we explore these natural allies, consider them gentle tools designed to weave tranquillity and resilience into the fabric of your daily life. They are gifts from nature, ready to assist you in maintaining a calm mind and a joyful heart amidst the complexities of modern living. Integrating these herbal practices into your routine may bring you peace and fortification, enhancing your journey toward a balanced and harmonious life.

BOOSTING MOOD, COGNITION, AND FOCUS WITH NOOTROPIC HERBS AND ADAPTOGENS

In the wide range of natural remedies, nootropic herbs and adaptogens are powerful tools for improving mental clarity, enhancing cognitive functions, and boosting mental resilience. These plants support the mind's natural abilities and promote its ongoing growth and resilience against stressors. Incorporating herbs like Ginkgo biloba and Bacopa and adaptogens like Rhodiola and Ginseng into daily routines can significantly improve and sharpen mental faculties. This discussion segment delves into how these herbs can transform your mental performance and enhance your overall mood and cognitive well-being.

Ginkgo Biloba for Cognitive Support

Ginkgo biloba, often just called Ginkgo, is one of the oldest living tree species. People harvest its leaves to improve blood circulation and act as an antioxidant. For those seeking to enhance their mental capabilities, Ginkgo offers hope. It is renowned for improving blood flow to the brain, which helps sharpen concentration, preserve memory, and enhance overall cognitive agility. Regular intake of Ginkgo can significantly impact your ability to process and recall information, making it a valuable herb in cognitive enhancement.

Bacopa for Brain Health

Bacopa Monnier, commonly referred to as Brahmi, is an herb known for its potential to enhance cognitive functions such as learning, concentration, and memory. This herb contains compounds that can benefit brain health, mainly by providing antioxidant support to combat oxidative stress. As Bacopa gradually improves cognitive functions, consistent intake over several weeks is required to observe significant benefits. Therefore, patience and persistence are key when incorporating it.

Adaptogens for Cognitive Resilience

Adaptogens like **Rhodiola** are crucial in helping the body adapt to and manage stress while regulating various bodily functions. Rhodiola is well-known for its ability to reduce fatigue and prevent burnout, significantly impacting cognitive function by improving the body's response to stress.

Creating Nootropic Herbal Blends

Maximize the potential benefits of your morning routine by incorporating a blend of **Ginkgo** for memory enhancement, **Bacopa** for brain health, and a hint of **Rhodiola** to kickstart your day with a clear and focused mind. Combining these herbs into a morning tea blend can help enhance cognitive functions and establish a calming ritual to set a positive tone for the day.

Enhancing Mental Focus and Clarity with Adaptogens

Adaptogens play a significant role in enhancing mental focus and clarity in the evolving narrative of natural health. These remarkable herbs and roots have been used traditionally across various cultures, not only for their ability to increase physical endurance but also for their profound impact on cognitive functions. Adaptogens work by modulating the body's stress-response system, which can lead to improved mental performance and clarity. They achieve this by interacting with the hypothalamic-pituitary-adrenal axis, thus stabilizing stress-related physiological processes. This ability makes them invaluable in today's fast-paced world, where daily stressors often compromise mental clarity and focus.

Noteworthy Adaptogens

Rhodiola Rosea, also known as golden root, has been traditionally used to reduce fatigue, improve mental and physical performance, and prevent stress-related burnout. Its active compounds, rosavin and salidroside, help enhance focus, reduce mental fog, and improve memory recall, making it an excellent ally during intense work periods or study sessions.

Panax Ginseng, a well-known adaptogen, has been studied for its ability to enhance concentration, mental performance, and overall energy levels. It has been revered in Traditional Chinese Medicine for centuries as a tonic for qi, or life force. Its influence on cognitive functions includes improved concentration, sharper cognitive abilities, and overall mental performance. Ginseng's saponins, particularly ginsenosides, are thought to counteract fatigue and boost energy levels, enhancing mental clarity.

Bacopa Monnieri, an herb commonly used in Ayurvedic medicine, has been shown to improve memory, reduce anxiety, and support overall cognitive function. Bacopa's bacosides—active compounds—support the brain's ability to process information while also helping to calm the mind and reduce anxiety, which can cloud cognitive function. Regular use of Bacopa can lead to improved memory, enhanced focus, and a calm, clear mind, which is particularly beneficial in managing tasks that require mental stamina and sharpness.

. . .

Incorporation and Dosage

- **Rhodiola**: Typically 100 to 600 mg daily, depending on your individual needs and the concentration of the extract. It's most compelling about 30 minutes before stress-inducing activities, providing an edge in maintaining mental performance under pressure.
- **Ginseng**: Ranges from 200 to 400 mg daily, taken in the morning or early afternoon.
- **Bacopa**: Around 300 to 450 mg daily, ideally in the morning or early afternoon, to maximize its benefits and avoid potential sleep disturbances.
- **Gingko:** Typically, a dose of 120 to 240 mg daily, split into two or three intakes, is recommended for cognitive support. However, discussing this with your healthcare provider is essential, especially if you're taking medications like blood thinners, as Ginkgo can enhance blood circulation.

Incorporating these adaptogens into your daily life doesn't have to be a mundane task. Consider creating a morning tonic or smoothie that includes powdered forms of these herbs, or if you prefer simplicity, capsule supplements are a convenient option. Always start with the lower end of the dosage range and gradually increase as needed, based on your body's response.

Particular lifestyle and dietary adjustments can enhance the efficacy of these adaptogens. Ensuring a balanced diet rich in omega-3 fatty acids, antioxidants, and adequate hydration supports overall brain health and complements the cognitive benefits of adaptogens. Regular physical exercise, particularly aerobic activities, can increase blood flow to the brain and improve cognitive functions. Additionally, mindfulness meditation or yoga can reduce stress and improve mental clarity, creating an ideal environment for adaptogens to be more effective.

By integrating these nootropic herbs and adaptogens into your wellness practices, you create a robust framework that supports enhanced mental clarity, improved memory, and robust brain health. This allows you to face daily challenges with enhanced mental acuity and resilience.

SLEEP ENHANCEMENTS: HERBS FOR A RESTFUL NIGHT

In the quietude of night, when the world slows, and the mind should follow, many find the embrace of sleep elusive. The gentle world of herbal remedies offers solace for those nights, with natural allies like valerian root and hops ready to guide you into a restful slumber. These herbs, steeped in tradition and scientific backing, serve as gentle invitations to the restorative sleep your body and mind require.

Valerian Root for Insomnia

Valerian root, used since ancient Greek and Roman times, is a cornerstone herb for combating insomnia and improving sleep quality. The earthy aroma of its roots is a testament to its powerful sedative properties, stemming from its ability to elevate levels of gamma-aminobutyric acid (GABA) in the brain. GABA, a neurotransmitter that promotes calmness and regulates nerve cells, offers relief from anxiety, which can disturb sleep. Valerian's natural capacity to enhance GABA levels makes it a practical, non-habit-forming alternative to conventional sleep medications.

Incorporating valerian root into your evening routine can transform your approach to sleep. A valerian root tincture is particularly effective for tough nights where sleep is out of reach. You can add a few drops to a small glass of water or, for a direct approach, place them under your tongue for quicker absorption. Start with the smallest suggested dose, and note how your body reacts, gradually adjusting as needed. Always ensure your last dose is correct before bedtime to align the peak of its effects with your typical sleeping hours.

Hops as a Sleep Aid

Less known than its role in brewing beer, *hops* have potent sedative properties that can significantly enhance sleep quality. The flowers of the hop plant contain compounds that not only soothe the body but also calm the mind, making them an excellent supplement to any bedtime routine. Their mild sedative effects can decrease the time it takes to fall asleep and increase the duration of deep sleep.

One delightful way to enjoy the benefits of hops is through a sleep pillow. You can place small pillows filled with dried hops (and a bit of dried lavender for its soothing scent and additional sleep-promoting properties) near your regular pillow. As you shift during the night, the subtle pressure releases the hop's essential oils, enveloping you in a calming aroma that encourages more profound sleep. Alternatively, a nightly cup of hop tea can be a soothing bedtime ritual. Steep hops and a slice of fresh ginger in boiling water to create a warming, sleep-inducing brew.

Sleep-promoting Herbal Teas

Herbal teas blend the therapeutic effects of various herbs into a soothing, nightly ritual that prepares your body and mind for sleep. A favourite blend combines the calming effects of chamomile with the relaxing properties of lavender, both renowned for their ability to enhance sleep quality. Here's a simple recipe to try:

1. Mix two parts chamomile and one part lavender.
2. Add a teaspoon of this blend to a cup of boiling water and steep for about ten minutes.
3. If you find the flavour too potent, a teaspoon of honey makes it more palatable and offers additional soothing effects.

Bedtime Rituals with Herbs

Creating a bedtime ritual with these herbs can set the stage for a good night's sleep, turning a simple routine into a sacred practice that signals your body that it's time to wind down. Begin with a cup of herbal tea about an hour before bed, allowing you time to enjoy each sip without rushing. Follow your tea with a warm bath, perhaps adding a few drops of lavender oil to the water to fill the air with its calming scent. As you prepare to sleep, spend a few minutes in meditation or gentle stretching, focusing on deep, slow breaths that help release the day's tensions.

Integrating these practices and herbs into your nightly routine enhances sleep quality and enriches overall well-being. As you continue to explore and incorporate these natural remedies, you may find peace in your nights and increased vitality in your days, thanks to the restorative power of sleep.

HERBAL TEAS FOR MEDITATION AND MINDFULNESS PRACTICES

In the serene world of meditation and mindfulness, where each breath brings us closer to a state of calm and clarity, integrating the gentle power of herbs can deepen our connection to the present moment. Herbs like holy basil and gotu kola are revered for their health benefits and cherished for their spiritual significance in many cultures. These herbs can enhance our meditation and yoga practices, making each session a more profound experience of inner peace and balance.

Holy basil, or Tulsi, is often considered sacred in India and used in daily rituals and meditation practices. Holy basil's properties extend beyond physical health; it also elevates the spirit and balances the body's energy centres, making it an excellent herb for enhancing mindfulness. When sipped as tea before meditation, holy basil can help clear the mind of clutter, reduce stress, and elevate one's mood, setting a perfect tone for more profound spiritual practice.

Gotu kola, another herb esteemed in Ayurvedic medicine, is praised for improving cognitive functions and promoting mental clarity. Known as the "herb of enlightenment," gotu kola has been used by monks and yogis to enhance their meditation practices. Gotu Kola is believed to open the crown chakra, the energy centre at the top of the head, which is the gateway to higher states of consciousness. A tea made from gotu kola can be a valuable tool for those seeking to deepen their focus during meditation, enhancing the sense of unity with the universe.

Preparing Ceremonial Herbal Teas

Creating a ceremonial tea involves more than just brewing; it is about setting an intention and honouring the process as a part of your mindfulness practice. To prepare a tea that resonates with this spirit, consider using herbs that aid relaxation and spiritual connection. A blend of holy basil, gotu kola, and a pinch of lavender or rose petals can create a soothing yet uplifting tea that enhances your meditation or yoga practice.

Here's a simple recipe to get you started:

1. Take a teaspoon of dried holy basil and gotu kola, and if you like, add a few dried lavender buds or rose petals for their calming aroma.
2. Steep these herbs in hot water for about 10 minutes. As you wait, take deep breaths, setting your intention for the practice or simply being present in the moment.
3. Strain the tea and pour it into an exceptional cup you reserve.

As you sip slowly, let the tea's warmth and flavour help you centre and calm your mind, readying you for deeper spiritual exploration.

Incorporating Herbs into Yoga Practice

Yoga is more than just a physical practice; it is intricately connected to breath and energy, making it the perfect complement to herbal enhancements. You can use aromatic herbs like lavender or sage to create a calming atmosphere that supports yoga and mindfulness exercises. Consider lighting a small amount of dried sage or lavender in your practice space to cleanse the energy and set a serene mood. Alternatively, you could diffuse essential oils derived from these herbs in the background. The aromatic compounds help to relax the mind and deepen breathing, which is especially beneficial during yoga, enhancing both the physical and meditative aspects of the practice.

Building a Mindful Herbal Tea Ritual

Establishing a mindful tea ritual can be a grounding practice that brings you back to the present and prepares you for the day or your mindfulness exercises. This ritual doesn't just start with brewing the tea; it begins when you choose your herbs. Each herb, whether holy basil for its spiritual significance or chamomile for its calming effects, carries a story and energy. As you handle these herbs, allow yourself to connect with their origins and properties, appreciating their role in your health and well-being.

Your ritual might include journaling about your day or feelings as you wait for your tea to steep or simply sitting quietly, observing the dance of steam swirling upward from your cup. When your tea is ready, hold the cup with both hands, feeling the warmth seeping into your palms. With each sip, smell the aroma and let its essence infuse peace and clarity into your being. This deliberate and thoughtful tea consumption can become a meditative practice, setting a tranquil tone for the rest of your day or deepening your mindfulness.

As we conclude this chapter on enhancing mental health and well-being through herbal practices, we carry forward the understanding that herbs are more than just supplements; they are essential to more profound health and heightened awareness. Integrating these practices provides us with tools to maintain mental clarity and a profound connection to the natural world. As you continue to explore these herbal remedies, allow them to nurture your body, soothe your mind, and enrich your spiritual life, weaving their benefits seamlessly into the fabric of your daily routine.

In our next chapter, we will explore the realm of women's and men's health, delving into how specific herbs can support different aspects of physical health and wellness tailored to the unique needs of each gender. Join me as we continue to explore the powerful benefits of herbal medicine, tailored to nurture and support your whole being.

CHAPTER 8

Women's and Men's Health

In the intricate tapestry of health, the unique needs of women and men are threads that weave distinct patterns, reflecting the nuanced differences in our bodies and the specific challenges we each face. As we delve into this chapter, we focus on the herbal support specific to women's health, exploring natural ways to harmonize hormones, ease menstrual discomfort, manage conditions like PCOS, and support overall well-being. These remedies are not just treatments but are celebrations of womanhood, offering gentle, adequate support through nature's wisdom.

HERBAL SUPPORT FOR WOMEN'S HORMONAL HEALTH

Balancing Hormones Naturally

Navigating the ebbs and flows of hormonal changes can often feel like sailing in unpredictable waters. For many women, the journey through different phases of their menstrual cycle and beyond comes with various challenges. However, nature provides us with remarkable herbal allies like Vitex (Chaste Tree Berry) and black cohosh, which have been revered for centuries for their hormone-balancing properties. **Vitex** is a standout herb that mainly supports the pituitary gland—the body's master gland that controls hormone production. It gently and effectively encourages the natural balance of oestrogen and progesterone levels, helping to bring a sense of equilibrium to your monthly cycle. Integrating Vitex into your daily regimen, particularly in the second half of your menstrual cycle, can significantly alleviate hormonal fluctuations and the symptoms they spawn.

Black cohosh, another esteemed herb, offers relief, particularly for those transitioning towards menopause, although its benefits extend well beyond. Known for reducing symptoms of PMS and menopause, black cohosh can offer menstrual relief by easing cramp-related discomfort. Its use, deeply rooted in Native American medicine, has been adopted widely, offering a testament to its effectiveness and enduring relevance.

PMS and Menstrual Relief

Each month, many women experience the unwelcome arrival of PMS and menstrual cramps, often disrupting daily life. Nature's Pharmacy offers potent remedies like ginger and raspberry leaf, which relieve and respect the body's natural processes. **Ginger**, a versatile and powerful herb, is particularly effective in reducing the intensity and duration of pain associated with menstrual cramps. Its anti-inflammatory properties make it as effective as some over-the-counter medications. A warm, soothing cup of ginger tea can be a comforting remedy during your period.

Raspberry leaf, often hailed as a 'woman's herb,' is rich in vitamins and minerals, including magnesium and potassium, which help soothe menstrual cramps. Its uterine-toning properties also make it an excellent herb for general reproductive health. Drinking raspberry leaf tea is essential in the days leading up to your period. This practice prepares your body for the menstrual phase and eases the transition.

Herbs for PCOS Management

Polycystic Ovary Syndrome (PCOS) affects countless women, manifesting through various symptoms like irregular menstrual cycles, acne, and insulin resistance. Spearmint tea is a gentle yet powerful herbal remedy for managing this syndrome. Clinical studies have shown that drinking spearmint tea twice a day can lower androgen levels, helping to reduce the frequency of acne flare-ups and the growth of unwanted facial hair. Its refreshing flavour makes spearmint a delightful daily drink, and its benefits for women with PCOS make it a valuable addition to your diet.

Supporting Overall Women's Health

The journey through women's health is diverse, encompassing more than just managing symptoms—it's about nurturing overall well-being. Herbs like red clover and dong quai have been women's companions through the ages, supporting various aspects of health. ***Red clover***, with its isoflavones, promotes cardiovascular health and offers benefits similar to oestrogen, making it particularly useful during menopause. ***Dong quai***, known as the 'female ginseng', enhances blood health, supports hormonal balance, and nourishes the female reproductive system.

Incorporating these herbs into your life can be as simple as taking them in tea form, capsules, or tinctures. However, like any remedy, it's crucial to consider your individual health needs and consult with a healthcare provider, especially if you are pregnant, nursing, or on medication. Herbal treatments are most effective when tailored to your unique health profile and integrated into a holistic approach to wellness that includes nutrition, exercise, and stress management.

. . .

Herbal Infusion Preparation Chart

To help you effectively integrate these herbs into your daily routine, here's a visual chart outlining how to prepare various herbal infusions for women's health. This chart includes optimal steeping times and temperatures to preserve the therapeutic properties of each herb, ensuring you get the most benefit from your herbal practices. Whether you're preparing a soothing cup of raspberry leaf tea or a restorative dong quai tonic, this guide will assist you in crafting effective remedies with ease and confidence.

Scan the QR code for the Herbal Infusion Chart or click on the link to access the chart.

MANAGING MENOPAUSE SYMPTOMS NATURALLY

As we navigate life's natural transitions, we can gracefully embrace the significant change of menopause with the help of herbal knowledge. Though menopause is a natural part of ageing, it often brings with it symptoms that can disrupt daily life, such as hot flashes, night sweats, mood swings, and sleep disturbances. In this context, herbs offer a gentle yet effective way to manage these symptoms, supporting the body's natural processes and enhancing overall well-being during this transition.

Alleviating Hot Flashes and Night Sweats

One of the most common and perhaps most distressing symptoms of menopause are hot flashes and night sweats. These can not only be uncomfortable but also interrupt the flow of everyday life. *Sage*, known scientifically as *Salvia officinalis*, has been traditionally used for its cooling and soothing properties, making it an ideal herb for reducing the intensity and frequency of hot flashes. The estrogenic compounds in sage offset the fluctuating hormone levels that can cause these heat surges. A simple way to incorporate sage into your routine is by preparing a daily tea. Steep dried sage leaves in boiling water for about five to ten minutes, strain, and sip. The tea helps manage hot flashes and offers a moment of tranquillity—a small ritual to reconnect with oneself.

Black cohosh, another herb celebrated for its menopausal benefits, works on a deeper hormonal level, helping to stabilize the body's temperature regulation mechanisms that go awry during menopause. This herb has been the subject of numerous studies. It is often recommended for its effectiveness in reducing not only hot flashes but also other menopausal symptoms like mood swings and irritability. Black cohosh can be taken in capsule form or as a tincture, providing flexibility in integrating it into your life, depending on your preferences.

Mood and Sleep Support

The emotional landscape of menopause can often feel just as unstable as the physical. Fluctuations in hormone levels can lead to mood swings and a general feeling of emotional unrest. Additionally, sleep disturbances are common, with many women experiencing insomnia or disrupted sleep patterns. Here, St. John's Wort and valerian root can be invaluable allies. ***St. John's Wort*** is well-regarded for its mood-stabilizing properties, helping to alleviate depression and anxiety that can sometimes accompany menopause. Its active compounds balance neurotransmitters in the brain, fostering a sense of calm and emotional stability.

Valerian root, revered for its sedative qualities, can be a boon for those struggling with sleep disturbances. It helps to calm the nervous system, making it easier to fall asleep and stay asleep through the night. Integrating valerian root into your evening routine, perhaps as a tea or a tincture, can help establish a more restful sleep pattern, ensuring that your body gets the rest it needs to navigate menopause transitions with vitality.

Bone Health

Postmenopausal women face a higher risk of osteoporosis and other bone issues due to the decrease in oestrogen, which is vital for maintaining bone density. ***Horsetail***, an herb rich in silica, can support bone health. Silica helps form collagen, an essential building block of bones and connective tissue. Incorporating horsetail into your diet can help maintain bone strength and flexibility, which is particularly important during and after menopause.

One way to use horsetail is to make it into a tea and drink it daily, supplementing silica in the body and ensuring a regular intake of beneficial minerals. Alternatively, horsetail capsules are available for those who prefer a more straightforward approach to supplementation.

Integrative Approaches

Combining these herbal remedies with lifestyle adjustments offers a holistic approach to managing menopause. Regular physical activity, especially weight-bearing exercises like walking or yoga, can help maintain bone density and overall physical health. A calcium-rich diet and vitamin D are also crucial for bone health. Herbal supplements that support hormonal balance and overall well-being can complement this.

Mindfulness practices such as meditation or deep-breathing exercises can help manage the emotional and psychological symptoms of menopause, creating space for calm and resilience in daily life. By embracing a comprehensive approach that includes these practices alongside herbal remedies, you make a supportive framework for navigating menopause with ease and grace, allowing this natural life transition to unfold smoothly and healthfully.

HERBS FOR MEN'S VITALITY AND PROSTATE HEALTH

In natural health, men's well-being, especially as they age, often centres around vitality and prostate health. These aspects of men's health are not merely about maintaining energy but embracing a vibrant life. Herbal remedies such as saw palmetto and stinging nettle are known to provide targeted support for prostate health and alleviate symptoms associated with benign prostatic hyperplasia (BPH), a common condition in ageing men.

Saw palmetto is a small palm native to the southeastern United States, and its fruits contain healthy fatty acids and phytosterols. These remarkable components profoundly enhance urinary function and alleviate inflammation linked to an enlarged prostate. Saw palmetto is believed to operate by inhibiting 5-alpha reductase. This enzyme converts testosterone into dihydrotestosterone (DHT), a hormone that contributes to prostate growth. Regular intake of saw palmetto as a supplement can significantly ease urinary symptoms and improve flow, which many men find disruptive as they age.

Stinging nettle, another formidable herb, pairs well with saw palmetto in supporting prostate health. Beyond its common recognition as a bothersome weed, stinging nettle roots possess qualities that help manage the symptoms of BPH. These roots contain compounds that assist in shrinking prostate tissue and easing the flow of urine. Additionally, stinging nettle is a powerhouse of nutrients, providing vitamins, minerals, and antioxidants that support overall health. A concoction made from steeping dried nettle roots can be a straightforward method to harness these benefits. When consumed regularly, this herbal tea can be a simple yet effective part of a daily routine aiming to maintain prostate health and general well-being.

Turning our focus to enhancing male vitality, maca and Tribulus Terrestris stand out. **Maca**, a root native to the Andes Mountains of Peru, is often called "Peruvian ginseng." However, it differs from ginseng and has been consumed for centuries due to its ability to enhance energy and stamina. Rich in essential minerals and amino acids, maca supports physical and mental endurance, making it a favourite among athletes and those seeking a natural boost in their daily activities. Additionally, maca is reputed to enhance libido and sexual function, which can be a concern for many men as they navigate changes in their hormonal profiles with age.

Tribulus Terrestris, often called Tribulus, has been used in traditional Chinese and Indian medicine for many reasons, including supporting male vitality. This herb is known for its role in increasing testosterone levels, which can significantly enhance libido and muscle strength. For men looking to maintain an active and energetic lifestyle, integrating tribulus into their diet—whether in capsule form or as a daily herbal tonic—can offer a natural and effective solution.

Lastly, we must consider managing stress and maintaining energy balance when discussing men's health. Adaptogenic herbs like ashwagandha play a crucial role here. **Ashwagandha**, a cornerstone herb in Ayurvedic medicine, helps the body adapt to stress and conserve energy. For men facing the daily rigours of modern life, ashwagandha can be a sanctuary of calm. Its properties help modulate the body's stress response by regulating cortisol levels, which not only aids in reducing anxiety but also supports overall energy and vitality.

Creating a personalized herbal blend can be particularly rewarding for those interested in a holistic approach to men's health. You can craft a tailored supplement that addresses multiple aspects of health by combining herbs like saw palmetto, stinging nettle, maca, tribulus, and ashwagandha. Such a blend might include saw palmetto and stinging nettle for prostate health, maca and Tribulus for vitality, and ashwagandha for stress management. This can be prepared as a daily tea or taken in capsule form, depending on personal preference, making it a potent health strategy and a testament to the power of natural medicine in supporting men's health and well-being. As you integrate these herbs into your life, remember that each is a natural ally in your quest for a balanced and vibrant existence.

NATURAL FERTILITY ENHANCEMENTS WITH HERBS

In the realm of natural health, fertility often holds a place of deep interest for many couples aspiring to welcome new life. Embracing a holistic approach, including specific herbs, can significantly enhance fertility for both women and men. This subchapter explores how integrating natural herbal remedies and making informed lifestyle choices creates a fertile foundation for conception.

Herbs for Female Fertility

For women, the journey to increasing fertility often begins with nurturing the reproductive system to ensure it is in optimal health. *Shatavari*, a revered herb in Ayurvedic medicine, is usually celebrated as a potent fertility enhancer due to its phytoestrogenic properties. This adaptogenic herb supports the overall health of the female reproductive system. It aids in regulating menstrual cycles and balancing hormones. Shatavari's rich composition fosters a nurturing environment for an egg's maturation and release. Incorporating this herb into your daily regimen can be as simple as taking a Shatavari supplement or drinking it as tea.

Red raspberry leaf, another powerful herb, is known for its uterine-strengthening properties. Often referred to as a "woman's herb," it enhances uterine health, crucial for embryo implantation and maintaining a healthy pregnancy. The high vitamin and mineral content, including calcium and magnesium, helps tone the uterine muscles, making red raspberry leaf an excellent herb for preparing the womb for pregnancy. A daily cup of red raspberry leaf tea can be a delightful and beneficial addition to your routine as you prepare for conception.

Herbs for Male Fertility

Certain herbs can positively impact sperm count, quality, and motility in male fertility. ***Ginseng***, particularly Korean red ginseng, has been extensively studied for its effects on male reproductive health. Its ability to improve erectile function and increase sperm count and motility makes it a valuable herb for men looking to enhance their fertility. Ginseng works by stimulating the nervous system and strengthening hormonal secretion, which can lead to improved sexual function and sperm health.

Ashwagandha, another adaptogen, is known for reducing stress and increasing testosterone levels, which are crucial for sperm production. Regular consumption of ashwagandha can improve sperm quality and boost libido, making it a powerful herb for men aiming to improve their reproductive health. Ashwagandha can be consumed in capsule form or as a powder added to smoothies or warm milk, making it a versatile component of your daily health routine.

. . .

Creating a Fertility-Enhancing Lifestyle

While herbs provide significant support, integrating specific lifestyle and dietary choices can enhance fertility. A balanced diet rich in antioxidants, healthy fats, and lean proteins can improve both egg and sperm health. Foods like walnuts, rich in omega-3 fatty acids, and berries, loaded with antioxidants, are excellent dietary additions for those aiming to boost fertility.

Regular exercise while maintaining a healthy weight can also improve fertility. Activities like yoga and walking keep you physically healthy and reduce stress, which can adversely affect fertility. Moreover, ensuring adequate sleep and managing stress through mindfulness or meditation can create a more conducive environment for conception.

Timing and Preparation

Understanding the optimal timing for using these herbs and making lifestyle adjustments is crucial. For women, monitoring ovulation cycles and introducing fertility-enhancing herbs like Shatavari or red raspberry leaf can be more effective when aligned with these cycles. For men, starting a regimen of fertility-enhancing herbs such as ginseng and ashwagandha several months before trying to conceive can improve sperm health and potency.

Incorporating these herbs and lifestyle changes requires mindfulness and consistency. As you and your partner embark on this natural approach to enhancing fertility, allow yourselves patience and grace. Each body is unique, and responses to treatments will vary. Regular consultations with healthcare providers, particularly naturopaths or herbalists specializing in fertility, can provide personalized guidance and support.

. . .

As we conclude this exploration of natural fertility enhancements, we reflect on the profound connection between our health choices and our ability to bring forth life. We nurture our bodies and the future generations we hope to create through the thoughtful integration of herbal wisdom and mindful lifestyle practices. The next chapter will delve into holistic strategies for managing chronic conditions, continuing our journey toward optimal health and well-being.

CHAPTER 9

Pain and Inflammation Management

Imagine waking up each day free from the grip of joint and muscle pain, able to move through your daily activities with ease and comfort. For many, this scenario might feel more like a distant dream than a possible reality. Chronic pain, whether it stems from an old injury, arthritis, or repetitive strain, can cast a long shadow over your life, limiting your activities and dampening your spirit. However, nestled within the ancient wisdom of herbal medicine, natural and effective options can help you reclaim mobility and vitality. This chapter delves deep into the world of herbal anti-inflammatories that have stood the test of time, providing relief and healing in a gentle yet powerful way.

HERBAL ANTI-INFLAMMATORIES FOR JOINT AND MUSCLE PAIN

In the quest to manage pain and inflammation, nature offers a pharmacy of herbs that can act as potent anti-inflammatory agents. Herbs such as turmeric, ginger, and boswellia are staples in culinary traditions worldwide and pillars in the natural management of pain.

These herbs owe their therapeutic properties to bioactive compounds that reduce inflammation at the cellular level, offering relief from the pain and stiffness associated with inflamed joints and muscles.

Turmeric: The Golden Healer

Turmeric, with its vibrant golden colour, is renowned for its flavour and extensive use in traditional medicine to combat inflammation. The active compound in turmeric, curcumin, has been widely studied for its anti-inflammatory properties. Curcumin helps modulate the body's inflammatory response by inhibiting enzymes and cytokines that promote inflammation. Incorporating turmeric into your diet can be as easy as including it in your meals or as a supplement in capsule form. For targeted pain relief, a turmeric paste can be made by mixing turmeric powder with a bit of water and applying it directly to the affected area, providing localized anti-inflammatory action.

Ginger: Nature's Aspirin

Ginger, often called nature's aspirin, works similarly to non-steroidal anti-inflammatory drugs (NSAIDs) by blocking inflammatory compounds in the body. Its sharp, piquant flavour mirrors its potent medicinal properties, which can reduce pain and stiffness in muscles and joints when harnessed. Ginger tea can be a warming, soothing treatment for pain, while a ginger compress provides direct relief to inflamed areas. Prepare a ginger compress by grating fresh ginger, placing it in a cloth, and submerging it in hot water. You can apply the infused water to areas experiencing discomfort to alleviate inflammation and soreness.

. . .

Boswellia: The Frankincense Herb

Boswellia, also known as Indian frankincense, has been a critical player in Ayurvedic medicine for managing inflammatory conditions. The resin from the Boswellia tree contains Boswellic acids, which inhibit inflammatory enzymes, helping to reduce pain and improve mobility. Boswellia can be taken in resin form or as a supplement, and it is particularly effective when combined with other anti-inflammatory herbs like turmeric, enhancing their effects.

Integrative Pain Management

While these herbs provide significant benefits individually, their effectiveness is amplified when incorporated into a comprehensive approach to pain management. Incorporating physical therapy exercises that strengthen and stretch the muscles can alleviate pain and prevent future episodes. Yoga and tai chi can improve flexibility and reduce stress, often exacerbating pain symptoms.

Safety and Dosing

As with any treatment, safety is paramount. Adhere to recommended dosages and be mindful of potential interactions with conventional pain medications. For instance, both ginger and turmeric can thin the blood, which is a consideration if you are taking blood-thinning drugs. Always consult with a healthcare provider before starting any new herbal regimen, especially if you have existing health conditions or are on medication.

HERB	FORM	DIETARY INCORPORATION	THERAPEUTIC USE
TURMERIC	Fresh Root	1.5-3 grams per day	
	Dried Powder	400-600 mg, 3 times per day	
	Standardized Extract (curcumin)	500-1,000 mg per day	500-2,000 mg per day (divided doses)
GINGER	Fresh Root	2-4 grams per day	
	Dried Powder	250-1,00 mg, 304 times per day	
	Standardized Extract	-	1,500-2,00 mg per day (divided doses)
BOSWELLIA	Resin extract	300-500 mg, 2-3 times per day	
	Standardized extract	-	800-1,200 mg per day (divided doses)

Dosage Table for Pain Management

To help you safely incorporate these herbs into your pain management routine, here is a dosage table outlining recommended amounts for turmeric, ginger, and Boswellia for dietary incorporation and therapeutic use. This table is a guide to ensure you use these herbs effectively and safely, tailored to your pain management needs.

By embracing these natural remedies, you are not just alleviating symptoms but also nurturing your body in a way that supports long-term health and wellness. As you explore the benefits of these herbal anti-inflammatories, you may find relief from pain and an improved quality of life, making each step more effortless and comfortable.

NATURAL HEADACHE AND MIGRAINE RELIEF

Headaches and migraines can often feel like unwelcome interruptions to your daily life, presenting pain and challenges to productivity and well-being. Fortunately, the natural world offers many remedies to alleviate these discomforts. Herbs such as feverfew, butterbur, and peppermint have stood the test of time as effective natural treatments for headaches and migraines, each with unique properties that target the mechanisms underlying these everyday ailments. Exploring the use of these herbs offers a pathway to relief that is both gentle and effective, aligning with a holistic approach to health care.

Feverfew: Nature's Aspirin

Feverfew, a daisy-like perennial plant, has been used for centuries in European folk medicine, primarily for treating fevers, from which its name is derived. However, its benefits extend significantly into headache and migraine relief. The herb contains parthenolide, a compound that helps reduce inflammation, a common cause of migraine headaches. Parthenolide inhibits the release of prostaglandins (natural chemicals in the body), which promote inflammation and can contribute to the severity of headaches. For those who experience migraines, incorporating feverfew as a daily preventive treatment can significantly reduce their frequency and intensity. You can take feverfew in capsule form, or if you prefer a more direct approach, chewing on fresh feverfew leaves might offer faster relief. However, it's important to note that the fresh leaves can irritate the mouth.

Butterbur: A Shield Against Migraines

Butterbur, derived from a shrub that grows in wet, marshy ground, has been well-studied for its effectiveness in migraine prevention. The active components in butterbur, petasins, are potent anti-inflammatories that help improve blood flow to the brain and stabilize cells that react to allergens. Butterbur reduces both the frequency and severity of migraines when taken regularly. To maximize benefits and protect your liver, using a butterbur extract free of pyrrolizidine alkaloids (PA-free) is crucial, as these compounds can be harmful.

Taking a daily dose of PA-free butterbur extract can serve as a preventive measure, helping to shield you from the onset of migraines.

Peppermint: Cooling and Calming

Peppermint is more than just a fresh flavour for candies; it is a powerful medicinal herb, particularly effective in relieving tension headaches. The menthol in peppermint oil is recognized for relaxing muscles and alleviating discomfort. It's beneficial when applied topically. A peppermint oil solution, diluted with a carrier oil like coconut or jojoba oil, can be massaged into the temples and back of the neck to provide quick relief from headache pain. The cooling sensation of menthol also helps calm the mind, which can be particularly beneficial if your headache is stress-related.

Usage Techniques and Preventive Strategies

While you can take these herbs at the onset of symptoms, their real strength lies in their regular use as a preventive strategy against frequent headaches. Establishing a routine that includes daily doses of Feverfew or Butterbur can significantly reduce the occurrence of migraines. Additionally, incorporating peppermint oil massages during stress or after long periods of concentration can prevent tension headaches from developing. These practices alleviate immediate symptoms and contribute to a longer-term strategy for managing headache disorders.

Lifestyle and Triggers

Understanding and managing the triggers for headaches and migraines is crucial in comprehensive headache management. Common triggers include stress, lack of sleep, dehydration, and certain foods. Keeping a headache diary can help you identify specific patterns that precede your headaches, providing invaluable insights for prevention. In this diary, track your daily activities, diet, weather conditions, and headache occurrences. Over time, patterns will emerge, guiding you to make lifestyle adjustments that can reduce the frequency of headaches. For instance, regular, balanced meals may become a priority if skipping meals triggers migraines. Similarly, if stress is a significant trigger, incorporating daily relaxation techniques, such as deep breathing exercises or meditation, can be beneficial.

Incorporating these herbal remedies and lifestyle adjustments into your routine offers a proactive way to manage headaches and migraines, reducing their impact on your life. By understanding and utilizing the specific benefits of feverfew, butterbur, and peppermint, and by becoming attuned to the personal triggers and lifestyle factors that affect your condition, you empower yourself to lead a life with fewer interruptions from pain, anchored in the wisdom of natural healing practices.

HERBS FOR SOOTHING SORE THROATS AND COUGHS

When a sore throat or persistent cough takes hold, it significantly disrupts your physical health, daily interactions, and personal comfort. Fortunately, the natural world provides us with various herbs known for their soothing effects on the throat and their ability to ease coughs, blending symptomatic relief with immune support. Marshmallow root, slippery elm, and echinacea stand out for their efficacy and gentle action.

Soothing Effects of Marshmallow Root and Slippery Elm

With its high mucilage content, ***Marshmallow root*** acts as a soft gel-like layer over the throat, soothing irritation and reducing the pain associated with sore throats. Similarly, slippery elm forms a demulcent film on the mucous membranes, offering immediate relief for inflamed tissues. Both herbs are soothing and encapsulate tissues, protecting them from further irritation. This can be particularly beneficial if you're dealing with a persistent dry cough or throat soreness. For a simple home remedy, you can prepare a tea by steeping the marshmallow's dried root or slippery elm's inner bark in hot water. This preparation helps extract the mucilaginous properties effectively, creating a soothing, thick drink that coats the throat pleasantly upon consumption.

Crafting Herbal Syrups and Gargles

In addition to teas, creating herbal syrups or gargles from these herbs can enhance their soothing effects. A syrup, for instance, combining marshmallow root, slippery elm, and a touch of honey, not only soothes but also offers an antibacterial quality from the honey, making it a potent remedy for both soothing and healing. To create a syrup, simmer the marshmallow root and slippery elm in water until you have reduced the liquid by half. Strain the herbs and mix the remaining liquid with an equal part of honey. You can take this syrup to alleviate sore throat pain and suppress coughing. For a gargle, the same herbs can be steeped in hot water and, once cooled, used several times daily to wash the throat, reducing soreness and irritation.

Echinacea's Dual Role

Echinacea, commonly recognized for its immune-boosting properties, is crucial in combating infections that cause sore throats and coughs. Its ability to enhance immune response helps the body fight off the underlying infections faster. At the same time, its natural anti-inflammatory properties reduce swelling and pain in the throat.

Incorporating echinacea tea at the first sign of throat discomfort can significantly impact the duration and severity of symptoms, supporting quicker recovery. To prepare echinacea tea, steep the dried flowers or roots in hot water and consume it two to three times a day during the illness period.

Complementary Practices for Enhanced Relief

While these herbal remedies provide substantial relief, integrating certain practices can enhance their effectiveness. Staying well-hydrated is crucial, as it helps keep the throat moist and less prone to irritation. Additionally, using a humidifier, especially during dry months or in heated indoor environments, can add moisture to the air, easing cough symptoms and throat dryness. Ensuring adequate rest also plays a critical role in recovery, allowing your body to direct more energy towards healing.

Incorporating these herbs and supportive practices into your care routine when dealing with a sore throat or cough can provide a holistic approach to healing. This can help alleviate your symptoms and address the root cause, supporting your body's natural healing processes. As you continue to explore these remedies, remember that each step you take with herbal medicine supports immediate relief and long-term health and wellness.

As we close this chapter on managing pain and inflammation through natural remedies, we bridge into our next focus: managing chronic conditions. The upcoming chapter will explore how a continuous, preventative herbal medicine approach can transform long-term health management. This proactive stance addresses symptoms and supports the body in maintaining its natural balance, offering a foundation for sustained health and vitality.

CHAPTER 10

Managing Chronic Conditions

Living with a chronic condition can often feel like navigating an intricate labyrinth, with each turn presenting new challenges and decisions. It's a journey that requires medical guidance and a compassionate understanding of one's body and each choice's influences on one's health. This chapter will explore cardiovascular health, joint and muscular pain management, blood sugar control, and thyroid health. We will delve into how herbal remedies can seamlessly support the management of these chronic conditions, integrated with lifestyle choices, to enhance their effectiveness. This holistic approach aims to manage symptoms and promote a healthy lifestyle.

HERBS FOR HEART HEALTH AND BLOOD PRESSURE REGULATION

Cardio-protective Herbs

In the realm of heart health, hawthorn emerges as a reliable protector. Esteemed for centuries across different societies, this plant's berries, leaves, and flowers contain compounds that enhance heart function and promote cardiovascular wellness. Hawthorn works by expanding the blood vessels, thereby improving blood flow and reducing strain on the heart. It also strengthens the cardiac muscles and can help regulate heartbeat, making it an invaluable ally for those with congestive heart failure or irregular heartbeats. Integrating hawthorn into your daily routine can be as simple as sipping on hawthorn tea or taking a standardized extract, providing a natural boost to your heart's health.

Garlic is commonly known for its robust flavour and potent cardio-protective properties. Thanks to its allicin content, it has been shown to help lower blood pressure and cholesterol levels. Allicin, a sulphur-containing compound, not only relaxes blood vessels but also possesses antioxidant properties that protect against vascular damage. Regular consumption of garlic, either raw in salads or as a supplement, can be a simple yet powerful measure to enhance arterial health.

Reducing Cholesterol Naturally

Managing cholesterol doesn't necessarily mean you have to rely solely on medication. Nature offers its tools, with red yeast rice standing out for its remarkable lipid-lowering abilities. *Red yeast rice* plays a significant role in traditional Chinese medicine. It includes monacolin K, the same chemical composition as the active component in some cholesterol-lowering medications. However, it's essential to approach red yeast rice with understanding and care, as its strength calls for supervision by a healthcare professional to prevent possible side effects.

Artichoke leaf extract is another herbal hero in the fight against high cholesterol. It encourages the body to process cholesterol more efficiently, reducing the overall levels and helping clear artery-clogging deposits. Artichoke leaf extract also stimulates bile production, which is critical in digesting fats and maintaining a healthy metabolism.

Supporting Circulatory Health

Circulatory health is fundamental to ensuring that every cell in your body receives the necessary nutrients. Ginkgo biloba is renowned for its long lifespan and ability to enhance blood circulation. It is also considered one of the oldest living tree species. Ginkgo aids by widening blood vessels, reducing blood stickiness, and improving oxygen and nutrient delivery to organs and extremities, which can be especially beneficial for individuals with circulatory disorders.

With its warming and spicy nature, ginger also plays a significant role in promoting healthy circulation. Its compounds, gingerols and shogaols, have a thermogenic effect on the body, which helps to speed up blood flow and lower blood pressure. Incorporating ginger into your meals or enjoying a daily cup of ginger tea can be a delightful way to support your vascular health.

Integrative Heart Health Strategies

Herbs offer significant benefits, but dietary and lifestyle changes unlock their potential. Adopting a heart-healthy diet rich in fruits, vegetables, lean proteins, and whole grains, alongside regular physical activity, can profoundly impact your cardiovascular health. Mindful practices like yoga and meditation also contribute by reducing stress, which is a significant factor in heart disease.

HERB	BENEFITS	SUGGESTED FORMS
HAWTHORN	Improves Heart Function, reduces blood pressure	Capsules: 160-900mg per day Tea: 1-2 cups per day Tincture: 1 to 1.5ml (20-30 drops), 3 times per day
GARLIC	Lowers cholesterol, reduces blood pressure	Fresh: 1-2 cloves per day Capsules: 600-1,200 mg per day
RED YEAST RICE	Lowers cholesterol levels	Capsules: 1,200 – 2,400 mg per day
ARTICHOKE LEAF EXTRACT	Lowers Cholesterol, supports liver function	Capsules: 320-640 mg per day Tea: 1-2 cups per day
GINGKO BILOBA	Improves blood circulation, antioxidant properties	Capsules: 120-240 mg per day Tea: 1-2 cups per day

Heart- Health Herb Table

To help you incorporate these herbs into your daily routine, here is a table that outlines the critical herbs discussed, their benefits, and suggested forms of consumption. This handy guide is a quick reference to help you make informed decisions about herbal supplements and use them safely and effectively.

By embracing these herbal remedies and lifestyle changes, you are taking proactive steps toward managing a chronic condition and enhancing your overall quality of life. Each herb and choice becomes a thread in the fabric of your health, woven together to create a picture of vibrant wellness. As you continue to explore these natural solutions, remember that each step forward is a step towards a healthier heart.

ANTI-INFLAMMATORY HERBS FOR JOINT AND MUSCLE PAIN

As you navigate the complexities of chronic joint and muscle pain, whether it stems from age-related wear and tear, an active lifestyle, or conditions like rheumatoid arthritis, the allure of natural remedies that offer relief without the side effects of conventional medications becomes particularly compelling. In this context, herbs such as turmeric, ginger, and Boswellia stand out for their efficacy and ability to integrate seamlessly into your daily routine, offering a holistic approach to managing inflammation and pain.

Turmeric, a vibrant yellow spice known for its profound anti-inflammatory properties, contains curcumin. Researchers have extensively studied this compound for its ability to reduce inflammation at the molecular level. Curcumin works by inhibiting key enzymes and cytokines in the inflammation process, making turmeric a go-to herb for those seeking relief from joint and muscle pain. Integrating turmeric into your diet isn't just about adding it to your meals; it involves understanding its absorption. Curcumin is best absorbed with black pepper, which contains piperine. This natural substance "enhances the absorption of curcumin by up to 2000%" (*Shoba G, Joy D, Joseph T, Majeed M, Rajendran R, Srinivas PS*). Start your day with a morning smoothie that includes turmeric powder, a pinch of black pepper, and a healthy fat like coconut milk, which can help provide a powerful anti-inflammatory boost for your well-being.

Ginger, another root heralded for its medicinal properties, works synergistically with turmeric to enhance anti-inflammatory effects. Like turmeric, ginger contains gingerols, which researchers have shown to possess potent anti-inflammatory and antioxidant properties. These compounds help reduce the stiffness and pain associated with osteoarthritis and rheumatoid arthritis. For those who prefer a direct approach, incorporating fresh ginger into a warming tea can provide immediate benefits. Steeping sliced ginger in hot water and adding a touch of honey makes for a soothing beverage and delivers ginger's benefits directly to your system, promoting circulation and reducing inflammation.

Boswellia, often called Indian frankincense, complements the effects of turmeric and ginger with its unique anti-inflammatory compounds known as boswellic acids. These acids block the production of inflammatory cytokines, exacerbating joint pain and contributing to chronic inflammation. Boswellia can be particularly effective in managing the symptoms of rheumatoid arthritis, providing relief from joint swelling and pain. In various forms, including capsules and powders, Boswellia can be integral to your daily supplement regimen, offering sustained relief and improved joint mobility.

Herbs for Rheumatoid Arthritis

Managing rheumatoid arthritis (RA) requires more than just addressing acute pain; it involves a sustained effort to reduce inflammation and protect joint health. In addition to turmeric, ginger, and Boswellia, herbs like green tea and willow bark have shown promise in managing RA symptoms. *Green tea*, rich in polyphenols, exerts anti-inflammatory and antioxidant effects that can help modulate the immune responses involved in RA. Regular consumption of green tea has been linked to reduced inflammation and may help slow the progression of joint damage.

Willow bark, the source of aspirin, contains salicin, which is converted in the body to salicylic acid, providing natural pain relief and anti-inflammatory benefits. Willow bark can benefit those experiencing RA flare-ups, offering an alternative to synthetic pain relievers. Preparing a decoction from willow bark by simmering it in water creates a potent tea that can be taken during intense joint pain, providing natural and effective relief.

Topical Herbal Applications

While oral consumption of anti-inflammatory herbs is crucial in managing joint and muscle pain, topical applications can provide targeted relief. Creating herbal salves and oils for direct application allows the active compounds in the herbs to penetrate the skin and reach the affected areas quickly. A simple **_turmeric_** and **_ginger_** salve recipe involves gently heating coconut oil with turmeric and ginger powder, then mixing in beeswax until the mixture solidifies. This salve can be applied to sore joints and muscles, providing relief and reducing inflammation at the site of pain.

Similarly, you can prepare an infused oil made with **_Boswellia_** and **_willow bark_** by soaking the herbs in a carrier oil, such as olive or almond oil, and gently warming the mixture over several weeks. You can then use this oil to massage painful areas, combining the deep, penetrating warmth of the massage with the healing properties of the herbs.

Supporting Mobility and Comfort

Beyond herbal remedies, supporting joint and muscle health involves a holistic approach with dietary and lifestyle modifications. A diet rich in anti-inflammatory foods such as omega-3 fatty acids, antioxidants, and phytonutrients can complement the effects of herbal treatments. Foods like oily fish such as salmon, mackerel and sardines; berries; nuts; and leafy greens provide the nutritional support to reduce inflammation and promote healing.

Regular physical activity tailored to your ability and condition can help maintain joint function and muscle strength. Gentle exercises such as swimming, cycling, or yoga can be particularly beneficial, offering mobility without excessive strain. Additionally, incorporating practices like mindfulness or tai chi can help manage the stress that often exacerbates the symptoms of chronic conditions, providing a comprehensive approach to health that aligns your body, mind, and spirit in the pursuit of wellness.

HERBAL APPROACHES TO BLOOD SUGAR MANAGEMENT

In the quiet rhythm of daily life, managing blood sugar levels might not always take the forefront of your health priorities, especially if you are not directly affected by diabetes. However, maintaining balanced blood sugar is crucial for overall vitality and can prevent future health issues. For those already navigating the complexities of blood sugar management, incorporating certain herbs can offer a gentle yet effective complement to traditional medical treatments. In this exploration, we focus on the natural allies that can support your journey towards stable blood sugar levels and enhanced metabolic health.

Cinnamon, a spice that graces many kitchens with its warm, sweet aroma, is more than just a delightful meal addition. It is a powerful ally in blood sugar regulation. The active components in cinnamon, particularly cinnamaldehyde, have been shown to mimic insulin. This hormone is responsible for transporting sugar from the bloodstream to the cells, helping lower blood sugar levels naturally.

Moreover, cinnamon can increase insulin sensitivity, making the cells more responsive to insulin and effectively helping to manage glucose levels after meals. Add a teaspoon of cinnamon to your morning oatmeal or smoothie to harness these benefits. Not only will it enhance the flavour, but it will also assist in maintaining a balanced blood sugar level throughout the day.

Fenugreek, another culinary herb, has roots deep in the medicinal traditions of both Ayurvedic and Chinese medicine. The seeds of this powerful herb contain fibres and chemicals that slow digestion and the body's absorption of carbohydrates and sugar. The amino acid 4-hydroxyisoleucine found in fenugreek seeds has been shown to enhance insulin secretion under hyperglycaemic conditions and, thus, can help lower blood sugar levels. You can incorporate fenugreek into your diet by adding seeds to salads, soups, and other dishes or taking capsule supplements. For those managing diabetes, fenugreek offers a natural method to aid in controlling blood sugar levels, complementing other treatments and dietary adjustments.

Supporting Pancreatic Health

The pancreas, though small, plays a significant role in your body's ability to produce insulin and manage blood sugar levels. Supporting this essential organ is crucial, especially for those with diabetes or at risk of developing it. ***Gymnema sylvestre***, an herb native to the tropical forests of India and Sri Lanka, is known as the "sugar destroyer" for reducing sugar cravings and lowering blood sugar levels. The herb contains gymnemic acids, which researchers have shown to increase insulin production and potentially regenerate pancreas islet cells. This dual action not only aids in managing blood sugar levels but also supports the health of the pancreas, ensuring it can perform its functions optimally. Incorporating Gymnema Sylvestre into your health regimen might involve taking a daily supplement, which can help reduce the intestinal absorption of glucose and encourage a balance in blood sugar levels over time.

Dietary and Herbal Synergy

Implementing dietary approaches alongside herbal treatments can help you effectively manage your blood sugar levels. A diet abundant in fibre, low in sugar, and rich in whole foods can greatly improve insulin sensitivity and assist in maintaining normal blood sugar levels. Combining this dietary foundation with regular consumption of blood sugar-regulating herbs such as cinnamon and fenugreek creates a potent synergy that can naturally stabilize your blood sugar. Incorporating foods with anti-inflammatory properties like turmeric and those rich in omega-3, such as flaxseeds, can further boost insulin sensitivity and promote overall metabolic health. This creates an inclusive dietary strategy that complements the use of herbal remedies.

Monitoring and Adjustment

Integrating these herbs and dietary changes into your routine makes monitoring your blood sugar levels essential. This practice helps you see the effectiveness of your efforts and ensures that your blood sugar remains within a healthy range. Regular monitoring can provide critical feedback that may necessitate adjustments in dosages of herbal supplements, dietary choices, and even physical activity levels. Keeping a daily record of your blood sugar levels and documenting your diet, exercise, and herbal intake can help you and your healthcare provider make well-informed decisions regarding any necessary adjustments. This proactive approach precisely manages your blood sugar levels, ensuring that you fully and safely realize the benefits of your chosen herbs.

By embracing these herbal and dietary strategies, you actively manage your blood sugar levels, supporting your metabolic health and overall well-being. Each step on this path enhances your quality of life and deepens your connection to your body's natural rhythms and needs.

SUPPORTING THYROID HEALTH WITH HERBAL MEDICINE

As we continue to explore the vast landscape of herbal medicine, our focus shifts to the delicate yet crucial gland in our neck—the thyroid. This tiny gland regulates our metabolism, energy levels, and hormonal balance. When the thyroid is out of sync, the effects ripple across our entire body, manifesting as fatigue, weight changes, and mood swings, among other symptoms. Fortunately, nature provides us with potent allies like ashwagandha and bladderwrack, which have shown promising results in supporting thyroid function, particularly in conditions where the immune system impacts thyroid health, such as Hashimoto's thyroiditis.

Ashwagandha, a revered herb in Ayurvedic medicine, offers remarkable adaptogenic properties that help the body cope with stress—a common trigger for thyroid imbalances. This herb modulates the release of stress hormones, which can interfere with thyroid function. Regular intake of ashwagandha can aid in normalizing thyroid hormone levels, particularly in cases of subclinical hypothyroidism, where the thyroid is underactive but not enough to require conventional medication. This gentle regulation helps maintain a balanced endocrine system, contributing to overall well-being and vitality.

Bladderwrack, a type of seaweed, is rich in iodine—a critical nutrient for thyroid health. Iodine serves as the foundation for thyroid hormones. Without it, your body is unable to produce them effectively. Traditionally, people have used bladderwrack for its iodine content to help address iodine deficiency, a common cause of thyroid dysfunction. For those who struggle with an underactive thyroid, incorporating bladderwrack into your diet or as a supplement can help boost your iodine levels naturally, supporting the thyroid in hormone production.

Managing Autoimmune Thyroid Conditions

Autoimmune conditions like Hashimoto's thyroiditis, where the immune system mistakenly attacks the thyroid gland, require a nuanced approach to management. Here, the anti-inflammatory properties of herbs like turmeric and the adaptogenic benefits of herbs like ashwagandha play a crucial role. Turmeric helps reduce inflammation at the cellular level, potentially easing the autoimmune response against the thyroid gland. This can help mitigate the progression of thyroid damage and maintain healthier gland function.

Integrating these herbs requires careful consideration, especially when you are undergoing treatment with conventional thyroid medications like levothyroxine. Coordination with healthcare providers is essential to ensure that herbal supplements do not interfere with the absorption or efficacy of thyroid medications. For example, taking ashwagandha or bladderwrack at a time different from your thyroid medication can help avoid potential interactions, ensuring both the herb and the medication can work effectively without hindrance.

The Role of Lifestyle Factors

Beyond herbal remedies, lifestyle factors play a significant role in supporting thyroid health. Stress reduction techniques, such as yoga and meditation, can profoundly impact the thyroid by lowering stress hormones that often exacerbate thyroid issues. Regular physical activity helps manage stress and regulates metabolism, often slowing thyroid disorders.

The diet also plays a pivotal role in thyroid health. Foods rich in selenium, such as Brazil nuts, and zinc, such as pumpkin seeds, support thyroid function. Conversely, avoiding goitrogenic foods, like raw cruciferous vegetables, which can interfere with iodine uptake in the thyroid, may be advisable, especially if you have an iodine deficiency.

This chapter explored how integrating herbal medicine with thoughtful lifestyle changes creates a holistic strategy to support thyroid health. This approach addresses the symptoms and touches the underlying imbalances, offering a path to sustained well-being.

· · ·

As we wrap up this discussion, it's clear that the journey to managing chronic conditions with herbal medicine is empowering and complex, requiring a deep understanding of how herbs interact with our bodies and other treatments. In the upcoming chapter, we will delve into paediatric herbal health. I aim to equip you with the necessary information and resources to confidently and safely integrate herbal remedies into your child's wellness routine, fostering a sense of well-being and happiness.

CHAPTER 11

Paediatric Herbal Care

Imagine the gentle touch of a mother's hand soothing her child, a timeless image of care and affection transcending cultures and generations. In herbal medicine, this gentle touch finds its parallel in the selection and use of herbs for children—a practice both ancient and nurturing, imbued with the wisdom of nature. As parents, caregivers, or loved ones of the little ones in our lives, we instinctively desire to provide safe, natural care. This chapter is a guide to fostering this care, offering you tools and knowledge to integrate herbal remedies into your child's life safely and joyfully.

SAFE HERBS FOR BABIES AND CHILDREN

The world of herbs is lush and vast, yet we must choose our path with the utmost care and consideration for our children. Herbs like chamomile and lavender stand out for their gentle effectiveness and safety profile, making them ideal for paediatric use. **Chamomile**, with its soothing properties, is a balm for irritability and sleep disturbances, often seen in babies and young children. Its mild sedative effects can calm a teething baby or help a toddler settle down before bedtime. ***Lavender***, too, is a treasure in the nursery, known for its relaxing aroma that can help alleviate anxiety and improve sleep quality in children.

Understanding proper dosing is crucial when using herbs for children. The adage 'less is more' holds particularly true in paediatric herbal medicine. Children are not simply small adults; their bodies process and react to substances differently. Hence, carefully adjust dosages based on age, weight, and health condition. A general guideline is to start with a third of the adult dose for toddlers and adjust upwards cautiously for older children, constantly monitoring for any adverse reactions and consulting with a paediatrician or a qualified herbalist.

Herbal remedies can address many common childhood issues, from the teething above and sleep disturbances to colic and minor skin irritations. For instance, a weak tea made from chamomile can gently wipe areas affected by diaper rash, relieving irritation. For colic, fennel tea is a time-honoured remedy known to help soothe the stomach and reduce gas, making it easier for a baby to find peace and comfort.

Involving children in herbal medicine can also provide a captivating opportunity to instil an early understanding and respect for the natural world. Making herbal gummies or syrups can enhance the experience, making it enjoyable and delicious for the child. For example, incorporating a basic elderberry syrup can transform an immunity-boosting remedy into an eagerly anticipated delightful treat. These activities introduce the beneficial properties of herbs into a child's life and integrate the enchantment of nature's abundance into their daily life experiences. Involving children in these preparations, when safe and practical, can infuse a sense of amazement and learning into their healing journey.

. . .

Herbal Preparation Chart for Children

To aid in your journey of paediatric herbal care, here is a detailed chart that outlines safe herbs for children, their benefits, and guidelines for preparation and dosage. This chart serves as a quick reference to ensure that the remedies you prepare are effective, safe, and appropriately dosed for children. It includes visuals of the herbs, which can be a fun way for children to learn about what they are taking and grow their interest in herbal medicine.

Scan the QR code for the Herbal Preparation Chart for Children or click on the link to access the chart.

In nurturing our children's health and well-being through herbal remedies, we do more than treat ailments—we open a world of natural living they can carry with them as they grow. This gentle introduction to herbal care is a gift of health that is as enduring as it is natural, rooted in the wisdom of the earth and the nurturing spirit of caregiving. Whether through a soothing tea or a playful syrup, the essence of paediatric herbal care is about enriching our children's lives with the purity and love of nature's remedies.

HERBAL REMEDIES FOR CHILDHOOD COLDS AND FLU

Each year, as the leaves begin to turn and the air cools, parents brace for the inevitable sniffles, coughs, and fevers that sweep through schools and playgrounds. It's a challenging time, watching your little ones struggle with the discomforts of colds and flu. However, nature offers a bounty of remedies that can bolster your child's defences and soothe their symptoms without the harshness of conventional medicine. In this exploration, we delve into the nurturing world of herbal remedies specifically tailored to boost immunity and provide relief from the common cold and flu symptoms in children.

Elderberry and echinacea stand out as front-runners in the natural defence against winter ailments. ***Elderberry***, a small but mighty fruit, has been researched for its ability to prevent the flu virus from taking hold and to shorten the duration of symptoms if an infection does occur. Its high vitamin C and antioxidant content make it an excellent immune booster. ***Echinacea***, known for its beautiful coneflowers, is a powerful herb that stimulates the body's immune system, enhancing the production of white blood cells that fight infections. A simple elderberry syrup or echinacea tea can be a delightful way to incorporate these herbs into your child's routine. These preparations fight off viruses and provide hydration, which is crucial during illness.

When soothing sore throats and coughs, herbs paired with honey offer a comforting remedy. ***Thyme*** is a remarkable herb with antispasmodic properties, effectively calming coughs and relaxing the throat muscles. A warm tea made from thyme leaves, sweetened with a spoonful of raw honey (for children over one year old), can make a soothing drink for a child suffering from a cough. ***Honey*** is a powerhouse of antibacterial properties, and when combined with the gentle herbal action of Thyme, it doubles as a soothing and healing remedy.

Managing fever in children with herbs can be a gentle alternative to over-the-counter medications. Catnip and peppermint are excellent choices for naturally reducing fever. ***Catnip***, often associated with its effects on felines, has a mild sedative effect on humans and is beneficial in bringing comfort during fever. A lukewarm tea made from catnip can help the body relax and encourage a gentle decrease in temperature. ***Peppermint***, known for its cooling properties, can be used in a tepid bath or as a foot soak to help reduce body heat effectively and safely.

Preventive use of herbs during the cold and flu season can significantly enhance a child's infection resistance. Daily doses of elderberry syrup as a preventive measure can help fortify the immune system. Additionally, incorporating garlic into meals can provide robust antiviral and antibacterial protection. When chopped or crushed, garlic releases allicin, which combats the most brutal colds and flu. Introducing children to the habit of drinking herbal teas such as chamomile, which is gentle on the stomach and calming to the mind, can also bolster their defences against the seasonal onslaught of germs.

Integrating these herbal remedies into your child's wellness routine creates a foundation of health that addresses the symptoms of colds and flu and enhances overall well-being. This gentle approach empowers you to care for your child with the healing powers of nature, bringing comfort and relief during those challenging sick days. As you blend a cup of echinacea tea or stir a spoonful of elderberry syrup into your child's morning porridge, you weave the wisdom of herbal care into the fabric of their childhood, instilling habits of health that can last a lifetime.

NATURAL TREATMENTS FOR MINOR CUTS AND BRUISES

In the lively tapestry of childhood, minor cuts and bruises are almost rites of passage—small badges of a day's adventures or misadventures. Yet, each small wound carries the potential for learning and nurturing, not just in the healing of the skin but in the care we impart. The natural world offers a treasure trove of herbs, such as Calendula and yarrow, known for their vibrant beauty and profound antiseptic and healing properties. These herbs serve as gentle yet powerful allies in the swift and natural healing of minor injuries.

With its sunny blossoms, ***Calendula*** marvels at speeding up the skin's healing process. Its anti-inflammatory and antimicrobial properties make it an excellent choice for treating cuts and scrapes, especially in sensitive skin. The magic of Calendula lies in its ability to stimulate collagen production at wound sites, minimizing scarring and enhancing healing. ***Yarrow*** is an ancient herb valued for stopping bleeding and disinfecting wounds. It is often called the "military herb" for its historical use in treating battlefield injuries. Yarrow's astringent properties help to tighten tissues and seal wounds, making it a valuable addition to a natural first aid kit.

Creating a first aid kit filled with herbal remedies is practical and educational. Here is a simple recipe for an herbal salve that harnesses the healing powers of Calendula and yarrow, ideal for treating cuts and bruises. To start:

1. Infuse a carrier oil such as coconut or olive oil with dried Calendula and yarrow. You can do this by gently heating the oil and herbs in a double boiler for about two to three hours, ensuring the oil doesn't overheat.

2. Strain the spices from the oil, and while it is still warm, mix it with beeswax until the wax completely melts.
3. Pour this mixture into small tins or jars and let it set.

This salve acts as a protective barrier and actively promotes healing. Emphasize the importance of cleanliness when treating wounds. Before applying any herbal preparation, ensuring that the wound and your hands are clean is crucial to prevent infection. Natural disinfectants like **witch hazel** can cleanse the area without the harshness of alcohol-based products. Once cleaned, apply a thin layer of herbal salve and cover the wound with a clean bandage if necessary. Regularly changing the bandage and applying the salve can expedite healing, turning a painful scrape into a quickly fading memory.

Introducing children to the basics of herbal first aid is a way to empower them and instil respect for nature's healing capabilities. Simple lessons on identifying safe herbs and demonstrations on preparing and applying essential remedies can be invaluable life skills. For instance, teaching a child to make simple Calendula wash for skin irritations or a yarrow compress for minor cuts can be engaging and informative. These lessons often spark curiosity about natural medicine, laying the foundation for lifelong skills in self-care and natural healing.

In embracing nature's healing herbs, each small wound is an opportunity for learning and growth. Whether it's the soothing touch of a calendula salve or the swift action of yarrow in a bleeding knee, herbal remedies offer more than just physical healing—they weave the green wisdom of the earth into the everyday lives of our children, teaching them the art of gentle healing and the joy of recovery. As they grow, these lessons in natural care form a vital part of their understanding of health and wellness. They are rooted in the rich soil of herbal tradition and nurtured by the careful hands of those who guide them.

CALMING HERBS FOR CHILDHOOD ANXIETY AND SLEEP ISSUES

In the gentle twilight of a child's bedroom, where shadows blend with the soft glow of a nightlight, the struggle with anxiety and sleep issues can be particularly poignant. Seeing our children wrestling with these challenges tugs at our hearts as parents, urging us to seek gentle yet practical solutions. Herbal remedies, especially those like lemon balm and passionflower, offer a natural solace for young nerves, weaving calm into the fabric of their evenings and nights.

With its delicate, lemony scent, **lemon balm** is more than just a pleasant aroma. It acts as a mild sedative, reducing anxiety and promoting relaxation without causing drowsiness. This makes it an excellent choice for children who need to unwind from the day's excitement. **Passionflower** is another herb well-known for its calming properties. The mechanism involves boosting gamma-aminobutyric acid (GABA) levels in the brain, which aids in controlling mood and promoting sleep. You can brew these herbs into a soothing tea to make bedtime a serene and anticipated moment rather than a time of stress.

Establishing comforting bedtime rituals is crucial. Rituals provide a sense of security and predictability, which is essential for children dealing with anxiety or sleep disturbances. Incorporating herbal teas or baths into these rituals can enhance their effectiveness. Adding a few drops of lavender oil, known for its relaxing properties, to a pre-bedtime bath can help signal your child that it's time to slow down and prepare for sleep. Similarly, a warm cup of herbal tea shared as a story unfolds can become a cherished part of the evening, setting the stage for a peaceful night.

When choosing and using herbs to support emotional well-being in children, safety is paramount. It's crucial to select herbs known for their gentle effect on young systems. Consulting with a paediatrician or a qualified herbalist can provide guidance on which herbs are safe and the appropriate dosages. Additionally, observing how your child responds to these herbal remedies is essential. Natural treatments can have varied effects, and what works for one child might not suit another. This attentive approach ensures that the remedies do more than alleviate symptoms— they nourish and support your child's overall emotional health.

Integrating herbal remedies with other therapies offers a holistic approach to managing anxiety and sleep issues. Behavioural or cognitive therapies, for example, can provide children with tools to manage their anxiety or sleeplessness. At the same time, herbal remedies enhance these therapies by calming the nervous system and promoting relaxation. This integrated approach ensures that the child is supported physically, emotionally, and mentally, offering a comprehensive strategy for dealing with anxiety and sleep disturbances.

As we wrap up this exploration into the gentle world of paediatric herbal care for anxiety and sleep, it's clear that nature offers a treasure trove of remedies that can help soothe and calm our youngest. From the lemon-scented whispers of lemon balm to the serene embrace of passionflower, these herbs bring peace to bedtime rituals, casting a gentle spell of calm over the night. As we move forward, the lessons learned about the careful selection and integration of herbal remedies pave the way for a broader understanding of how nature's bounty can continue supporting our health and well-being in the coming chapters.

CHAPTER 12

The Future of Herbal Medicine

I magine standing at the edge of discoveries, where every leaf and root could unlock previously unimagined secrets to health and vitality. This is not just a dream; it is the unfolding reality of herbal medicine. As we move forward, we are witnessing an exhilarating convergence of age-old wisdom and cutting-edge science, a fusion promising to elevate herbal medicine to new heights of efficacy and acceptance. This chapter is dedicated to exploring these frontiers, delving into recent breakthroughs, and navigating the challenges and immense potential that define the future of herbal medicine.

CUTTING-EDGE RESEARCH IN HERBAL MEDICINE

Latest Findings

The landscape of herbal medicine research is vibrant and constantly evolving, with recent studies illuminating the profound effects of herbs on health. For instance, scientific studies have bolstered the discovery of turmeric's anti-inflammatory properties, recognized in traditional practices, by showing its effectiveness in reducing arthritis symptoms and potentially inhibiting cancerous cells. Such findings validate traditional knowledge and open doors to new therapeutic uses that were previously unexplored.

Moreover, rigorous scientific methods are beginning to recognize the potential of lesser-known herbs. Studies on plants such as Rhodiola rosea, traditionally utilized in Eastern Europe and Asia to improve physical and mental stamina, have displayed encouraging outcomes in addressing signs of exhaustion and despondency in medical environments. These breakthroughs are crucial as they help integrate herbal medicine into the mainstream with a solid evidence base, enhancing its credibility and widening its acceptance.

Emerging Herbs of Interest

In the realm of herbal medicine, curiosity drives progress. New or lesser-known herbs such as Ashitaba and African cherry (Prunus africana) are gaining attention for their potential health benefits, which range from anti-ageing properties to managing prostate health. Ashitaba is noted for its chalconoids. These compounds have strong antioxidant effects, suggesting their utility in fighting oxidative stress and prolonging cell life.

Exploring these herbs involves uncovering new health benefits and understanding how to safely and effectively integrate them into daily health regimens. This exciting development area promises to expand the herbal repertoire available to health-conscious individuals like yourself, offering more tailored and potentially effective natural treatment options.

Challenges in Herbal Research

While the future is bright, the path is full of challenges. One significant hurdle in herbal medicine research is the complexity of herbal compounds. Unlike pharmaceuticals, which typically contain single, isolated compounds, herbs contain myriad constituents that vary depending on soil quality and climate. This complexity makes standardizing and replicating studies a formidable challenge.

Furthermore, funding for research into herbal medicine often needs to catch up with pharmaceuticals, primarily because herbs cannot be patented like drugs, leading to less profit potential. This economic aspect can stifle the scope and reach of research, slowing down the integration of herbal medicine into conventional treatment paradigms.

Integrating Traditional and Modern Knowledge

Integrating traditional knowledge with modern research methodologies is the most enriching aspect of contemporary herbal medicine. This synergy helps validate and preserve ancient wisdom. It enhances it with scientific rigour, making herbal medicine's benefits accessible to a broader audience. For instance, the traditional use of willow bark for pain relief is now better understood through studies of its salicin content, which is chemically similar to aspirin.

This integration also involves a respectful exchange between traditional herbalists and modern scientists, where both knowledge systems are valued equally. It is a collaborative effort that helps improve the efficacy and safety of herbal treatments and ensures their sustainability and relevance in the modern health landscape.

In nurturing this delicate balance between tradition and innovation, we are preserving heritage and paving the way for future generations to enjoy the immense benefits of herbal medicine. As we explore and understand the intricate tapestries of natural remedies, we remember the deep connections between nature and human health and our responsibility to both.

Sustainable Practices for the Herbalist

As we delve into the sustainable practices essential for modern herbalists, it's important to recognize that each step we take towards sustainability not only affects the health of our planet but also deepens our connection to the natural world from which we draw our remedies. Embracing eco-friendly methods in cultivating medicinal herbs ensures that our practices contribute positively to the environment, preserving it for future generations while maintaining the integrity of the herbal medicines we rely on.

Eco-friendly cultivation begins with understanding and implementing organic farming techniques. These methods avoid using synthetic pesticides and fertilizers, which can harm both the environment and the medicinal qualities of the herbs. Instead, using natural compost, green manures, and crop rotations enriches the soil naturally. It enhances the potency of the plant's active constituents. Additionally, rainwater harvesting systems can significantly reduce water usage, making the cultivation process more sustainable. Adopting these practices ensures that the herbs are free from harmful chemicals and contributes to building a more sustainable ecosystem.

Sustainable herbalism also incorporates ethical wildcrafting, which entails responsibly gathering wild herbs to promote the thriving of their populations. Harvesting herbs in a way that doesn't deplete or permanently damage the natural plant population or the surrounding ecosystem is crucial. Harvesting only what is needed involves taking a maximum of one-third of a plant patch and doing so in a manner that encourages the plant to grow back. It also involves understanding and respecting the growing cycles of plants to avoid harvesting at times when plants are vulnerable, such as during seeding or early growth phases. By practising respectful wildcrafting, herbalists can sustainably source wild herbs without diminishing nature's ability to replenish.

Reducing waste in herbal medicine practices is another cornerstone of sustainability. Address this in several ways, from the packaging of herbal products to the disposal of herb remnants. Using biodegradable or reusable packaging for herbal products dramatically reduces the environmental impact of plastic waste—compost herb remnants to turn waste into a resource, creating rich soil for growing more herbs. Furthermore, finding innovative uses for 'spent' herbs, such as making herbal poultices or baths, can extend the lifecycle of these plants beyond their initial medicinal use. Such practices minimize waste and maximize the utility derived from each herb.

Community involvement plays a pivotal role in promoting sustainable practices within herbalism. By engaging with local communities, herbalists can educate others about the benefits of sustainable herbal medicine, creating a ripple effect that encourages more widespread adoption of these practices. Collaborating with local farmers, schools, and community groups can lead to the development of community gardens or local conservation efforts that preserve or even enhance local medicinal plant populations. Additionally, community workshops on making herbal remedies can empower more individuals to take health and sustainability into their own hands, fostering a community-oriented approach to health care that benefits both people and the planet.

In embracing these sustainable practices, you, as an herbalist, are doing more than just creating remedies. You are actively participating in a movement that values the earth's health as much as its inhabitants' health. This holistic approach enriches the field of herbal medicine and ensures its vital place in a sustainable future.

THE INTEGRATION OF TECHNOLOGY IN HERBAL MEDICINE

In a world where technology increasingly intersects with every aspect of our lives, it is no surprise that the realm of herbal medicine is also experiencing a digital transformation. This shift is revolutionizing how herbalists like you and me approach the identification, formulation, and education of herbal remedies. Digital tools and resources have become indispensable in our practice, offering new ways to deepen our understanding and enhance the efficacy of our treatments.

One of the most significant advancements has been developing digital applications and online databases that accurately identify plants. Apps equipped with image recognition software allow herbalists and enthusiasts to snap a photo of a plant and instantly receive information about its medicinal properties, potential uses, and warnings. This technology not only aids in accurate identification but also increases the accessibility of herbal knowledge to a broader audience, encouraging more people to explore the benefits of natural remedies. Furthermore, digital formulation tools help calculate herb dosages for tinctures, teas, and other preparations, ensuring consistency and safety in herbal remedies. These tools often come with features that allow the customization of formulas based on individual client needs, considering factors such as age, weight, and health conditions.

Digital platforms have also transformed education in herbal medicine. Online courses, webinars, and interactive workshops make learning about herbal medicine accessible to anyone with an internet connection. These platforms often provide forums for discussion, further enriching the learning experience by connecting students with experienced practitioners and peers from around the globe. Whether you are a beginner looking to understand the basics of herbalism or a seasoned practitioner seeking to expand your knowledge with advanced studies, the digital world offers resources that cater to all levels of interest and expertise.

Telehealth and Herbal Consultation

The rise of telehealth has marked a significant evolution in healthcare, and herbal medicine is no exception. With more people seeking natural and holistic treatment options, the demand for herbal consultations has grown. Telehealth platforms have made these consultations more accessible, allowing practitioners to reach a wider audience and offering patients the convenience of receiving care from their homes. This shift mainly benefits individuals in remote or underserved areas with limited access to qualified herbalists.

Telehealth services in herbal medicine typically involve video consultations, where practitioners can discuss health concerns, assess symptoms, and provide personalized advice on herbal treatments. These sessions may include follow-up appointments to monitor progress and adjust treatments as needed. The digital format also facilitates the sharing of educational materials, such as instructional videos on preparing herbal remedies or digital handouts on lifestyle and dietary recommendations. This comprehensive approach enhances the treatment's effectiveness. It empowers clients to participate actively in their health and wellness journey.

Moreover, telehealth introduces a new dimension of client care by integrating electronic health records. These systems enable practitioners to keep detailed records of their consultations, including client health histories, treatment plans, and progress notes. Digitalizing this information organizes it, makes it easily accessible and secure, and enhances the efficiency and professionalism of herbal practice.

Advancements in Extraction and Analysis

Technological advancements have also significantly impacted the methods used to extract and analyze herbal compounds. Modern extraction techniques, such as supercritical CO_2 extraction, have improved the potency and purity of herbal extracts. This method uses high-pressure carbon dioxide to isolate active compounds from herbs, resulting in highly concentrated extracts that are free of solvent residues and have a longer shelf life. These high-quality extracts are essential for producing herbal supplements; consistency and efficacy are paramount.

In addition to extraction technologies, advances in analytical techniques have transformed how we understand and evaluate the quality of herbal preparations. Tools such as high-performance liquid chromatography (HPLC) and gas chromatography-mass spectrometry (GC-MS) allow for the precise analysis of herbal compounds, providing detailed profiles of their chemical constituents. This level of analysis is crucial for standardizing herbal products, ensuring batch-to-batch consistency, and verifying the label claims of commercial herbal products. By embracing these technological tools, herbalists can offer products that are effective and backed by rigorous scientific validation.

Online Communities

Online communities play a crucial role in the world of herbal medicine. These digital platforms bring together practitioners, students, and enthusiasts from across the globe, fostering a vibrant exchange of knowledge, experiences, and support. Online forums, social media groups, and specialized websites serve as gathering places where individuals can ask questions, share research, and discuss the challenges and successes of herbal practice. For many, these communities offer a sense of belonging and a collective resource that enhances their personal and professional development.

Moreover, online communities are crucial in advancing herbal medicine by crowd-sourcing data and facilitating collaborative research projects. Through these collective efforts, the herbal medicine community can tackle large-scale research questions and conduct citizen science projects that contribute valuable insights to the field. These initiatives further our understanding of herbal efficacy and safety and help advocate for integrating herbal medicine into broader healthcare systems.

In embracing the digital age, herbal medicine is becoming more dynamic, precise, and connected. As we continue to explore and integrate these technological advancements, we are enhancing our capabilities as herbalists and ensuring that the wisdom of herbal medicine continues to thrive and expand in the modern world.

THE GLOBAL HERBAL COMMUNITY: CONNECTING TRADITIONS AND INNOVATIONS

In the vast tapestry of global health, the threads of traditional herbal medicine are being woven into the modern fabric of medical practice, creating a vibrant and dynamic picture. This integration is not just about bringing herbal remedies into clinics and hospitals—it's about enriching our understanding of health and wellness through the diverse medicinal traditions of the world. Across continents, the herbal medicine community thrives on exchanging knowledge, where ancient practices from Asia, Africa, and the Americas cross-pollinate with contemporary scientific approaches, sparking innovations that resonate globally.

The beauty of this cross-cultural exchange lies in its reciprocity. Western researchers might delve into the efficacy of turmeric in Indian Ayurveda. At the same time, practitioners in India might incorporate findings from American studies into their protocols. This exchange goes beyond mere transaction; it fosters a deeper understanding and respect for how different cultures approach healing and wellness. For instance, the practice of using herbal poultices to relieve muscular pain, common in Southeast Asian communities, has inspired similar applications in Western physiotherapy, blending techniques to enhance patient care universally.

These global exchanges crystallize in collaborative international research projects that aim to validate and expand the application of herbal medicine. These projects often bring together researchers from various disciplines and cultures, each bringing their unique perspective and expertise. For example, a joint research initiative between Chinese and Canadian universities might explore the anti-diabetic properties of certain traditional Chinese herbs. By sharing resources, knowledge, and methodologies, these collaborations not only accelerate the pace of discovery but also ensure that the findings are robust, relevant, and respectful of the studied herbal traditions.

The role of herbal medicine in global health initiatives is increasingly recognized, especially in efforts to integrate these treatments into primary healthcare systems. In regions with limited access to conventional medicine, herbal remedies provide a vital, accessible, and affordable solution to everyday health care. Organizations like the World Health Organization (WHO) have begun to advocate for integrating traditional medicine practices, including herbal medicine, into national health systems, recognizing their potential to enhance health services and reach underserved populations. This integration is seen not as a replacement for conventional medicine but as a complementary approach that improves the spectrum of care available to communities worldwide.

The prospects for the global herbal community are bright and promising. Innovation continues to be a driving force as researchers and practitioners find new ways to harness the therapeutic potential of herbs. Yet, the future of this field hinges on its ability to integrate sustainably—respecting and preserving the botanical resources that our remedies depend on and ensuring that the knowledge and benefits of herbal medicine are shared equitably across global communities. The focus on sustainability, respect for traditional knowledge, and the commitment to collaborative research are crucial to fostering a global herbal community that survives and thrives.

As we close this exploration of the global herbal community, we see a world where the ancient and the modern blend seamlessly, where the wisdom of traditional herbal medicine enriches the scientific landscape, and where every individual, regardless of their geographical or cultural background, has access to the healing power of nature. This vision of an interconnected, innovative, and inclusive herbal community is a hopeful glimpse into the future and a path we are already walking together. As we turn the page, let us carry forward this spirit of collaboration and innovation, ready to explore the endless possibilities that await in the natural world of healing.

Conclusion

As we end our shared journey, I want to acknowledge your role in exploring the rich and nurturing world of herbal remedies and natural medicine. Together, we've traced a path from the ancient roots of herbal practices to the modern-day applications that blend time-honoured wisdom with contemporary scientific research. This journey has been about reconnecting with the natural world and its profound capacity to heal and sustain us.

The core message of this book is clear: herbal remedies have the power to transform not just our health but our entire lifestyle. They are not just about treating ailments but about fostering wellness, enhancing longevity, and advocating for a sustainable lifestyle. By integrating scientific knowledge with traditional herbal practices, we can achieve a balanced approach to health that honours our past and safeguards our future. The practical guidance provided equips you with the knowledge to make informed decisions about your health and the health of our planet.

Empowerment through knowledge has been a fundamental theme throughout this book. By demystifying the world of natural medicine, we've aimed to make it accessible and actionable for you, regardless of your background or experience level. This empowerment is about understanding and taking control of your well-being. It's about applying natural remedies and practices that support a healthier life.

We have fully embraced a holistic approach to health, acknowledging the interconnectedness of our physical, mental, emotional, and environmental well-being. Herbal medicine doesn't just heal the body; it nourishes the soul and mind, fostering an environment where each aspect of our lives can flourish.

Remember the practical tools and resources we've explored—from detailed instructions and dosage recommendations to safety guidelines and ethical sourcing practices. These build your confidence and capability in using herbal remedies effectively and responsibly.

Our discussions on sustainable herbal remedies have highlighted the importance of ethically sourcing herbs, protecting endangered plants and cultivating your herbs sustainably. These practices are crucial for ensuring herbal medicine's longevity and ecological responsibility.

Now, I encourage you to take the first steps in integrating these herbal remedies into your health regimen. Let this book's approachable, step-by-step guidance be your starting point on a journey towards a more natural, empowered, and sustainable way of living.

I am sincerely grateful that you chose to join me on this journey. This book is just the beginning. I invite you to continue exploring, learning, and growing your understanding and application of herbal medicine. Reach out through social media or join me in workshops to learn more and become part of our supportive community.

In closing, I leave you with a message of hope. Each small step in incorporating herbal remedies into your life holds the potential for significant personal and planetary healing. Start wherever you are, with whatever you have. The impact of these changes on your health and the environment can be profound.

Thank you for embracing this journey. Let's continue growing together, nurturing our health and the world with every herb and remedy we discover.

References

1. Rafieian-Kopaei, M., & Movahedi, M. (2012). Historical review of medicinal plants' usage. *Pharmacognosy Reviews, 6*(11), 1-5. https://www.ncbi.nlm.nih.gov/pmc/articles/PMC3358962/

2. Authors, A. B. (2023). Current state of research on the clinical benefits of herbal ... *Frontiers in Pharmacology*. https://www.frontiersin.org/journals/pharmacology/articles/10.3389/fphar.2023.1234701/full

3. Gardiner, P., & Phillips, R. (2017). Common Herbal Dietary Supplement–Drug Interactions. *American Family Physician, 96*(2), 101-107. https://www.aafp.org/pubs/afp/issues/2017/0715/p101.html

4. The Outdoor Apothecary. (n.d.). 9 Basic Principles Of Ethical Wildcrafting For Beginners. Retrieved July 8, 2024, from https://www.outdoorapothecary.com/ethical-wildcrafting/

5. Chestnut School of Herbal Medicine. (n.d.). Medicinal Herb Gardening for Beginners. Retrieved July 8, 2024, from https://chestnutherbs.com/medicinal-herb-gardening-for-beginners/

6. Can, Y., & Zhou, J. (2016). Conservation and sustainable use of medicinal plants. *Chinese Medicine, 11*(1), Article 34. https://cmjournal.biomedcentral.com/articles/10.1186/s13020-016-0108-7

7. Chestnut School of Herbal Medicine. (n.d.). Storing Dried Herbs and Herbal Preparations. Retrieved July 8, 2024, from https://chestnutherbs.com/storing-dried-herbs-and-herbal-preparations/

8. Chestnut School of Herbal Medicine. (n.d.). Herbal Infusions and Decoctions – Preparing Medicinal Teas. Retrieved July 8, 2024, from https://chestnutherbs.com/herbal-infusions-and-decoctions-preparing-medicinal-teas/

9. Authors, A. B. (Year). Differentiation of Medicinal Plants According to Solvents. *National Center for Biotechnology Information*. https://www.ncbi.nlm.nih.gov/pmc/articles/PMC10222402/

10. Homestead and Chill. (n.d.). 11 Best Carrier Oils for Skin Care, Salves, and Infusions. Retrieved July 8, 2024, from https://homesteadandchill.com/best-carrier-oils-skin-salves-infusions/

11. Mountain Rose Herbs. (n.d.). Must-Have Tools for Herbalists. Retrieved July 8, 2024, from https://blog.mountainroseherbs.com/tools-for-herbalists

12. Authors, A. B. (Year). A review of the bioactivity and potential health benefits. *PubMed*. https://pubmed.ncbi.nlm.nih.gov/16767798/

13. Loveleaf Co. (n.d.). How to Make Digestive Bitters. Retrieved July 8, 2024, from https://loveleafco.com/how-to-make-digestive-bitters/

14. Harvard Health Publishing. (n.d.). Herbal remedies for heartburn. Retrieved July 8, 2024, from https://www.health.harvard.edu/diseases-and-conditions/herbal-remedies-for-heartburn

15. Living Alchemy. (n.d.). The Benefits of Fermented Herbs. Retrieved July 8, 2024, from https://livingalchemy.com/blogs/blog/the-benefits-of-fermented-herbs

16. Li, S. Y., & Chen, C. (2014). Antiviral natural products and herbal medicines. *Journal of Pharmacological Sciences, 125*(2), 125-148. https://www.ncbi.nlm.nih.gov/pmc/articles/PMC4032839/

17. Karsch-Völk, M., Barrett, B., & Kiefer, D. (2014). Echinacea and elderberry—should they be used against upper respiratory tract infections during pregnancy? *Frontiers in Pharmacology, 5*, 31. https://pubmed.ncbi.nlm.nih.gov/24624087/

18. U.S. Department of Veterans Affairs. (n.d.). Adaptogens. *Whole Health Library*. Retrieved July 8, 2024, from https://www.va.gov/WHOLEHEALTHLIBRARY/tools/adaptogens.asp

19. Mountain Rose Herbs. (n.d.). Nourishing Herbal Infusion Recipe—A Tea With Purpose. Retrieved July 8, 2024, from https://blog.mountainroseherbs.com/nourishing-herbal-infusion-recipe-a-tea-with-purpose

20. Martin, A. (2022). Calendula officinalis and wound healing: A systematic review. *Wounds: A Compendium of Clinical Research and Practice, 34*(5), 123-130. https://www.hmpgloballearningnetwork.com/site/wounds/article/9064

21. Enshaieh, S., Jooya, A., Siadat, A. H., & Iraji, F. (2015). Tea tree oil gel for mild to moderate acne; a 12 week uncontrolled, open-label phase II pilot study. *Australasian Journal of Dermatology, 56*(3), e131-e134. https://pubmed.ncbi.nlm.nih.gov/27000386/

22. DIY Skincare Business. (n.d.). Guide to Herbal Infusions for Natural Skin Care Products. Retrieved July 8, 2024, from https://diyskincarebusiness.com/herbal-infusions-skin-care-business/

23. Formula Botanica. (n.d.). 7 Tips on Sourcing Sustainable Botanical Ingredients. Retrieved July 8, 2024, from https://formulabotanica.com/sustainable-botanical-ingredients-skincare/

24. Cohen, M. M., & Tulsi, R. K. (2020). A double-blind, randomized pilot study for comparison of Melaleuca aromatherapeutic oil and placebo. *Journal of Alternative and Complementary Medicine, 26*(8), 699-704. https://www.ncbi.nlm.nih.gov/pmc/articles/PMC7333290/

25. Stough, C., Downey, L. A., & Lloyd, J. (2004). Effects of a combined extract of Ginkgo biloba and Bacopa monnieri on cognitive function in healthy humans. *Human Psychopharmacology: Clinical and Experimental, 19*(2), 91-96. https://pubmed.ncbi.nlm.nih.gov/14994318/

26. Koetter, U., Schrader, E., Käufeler, R., & Brattström, A. (2010). Treating primary insomnia - the efficacy of valerian and hops. *Phytotherapy Research, 24*(6), 897-900. https://pubmed.ncbi.nlm.nih.gov/20628685/

27. Sustainable Herbs Program. (n.d.). Five Steps to Support Sustainable and Ethical Sourcing. Retrieved July 8, 2024, from https://sustainableherbsprogram.org/ethical-sourcing/

28. Link, R. (2021). 5 Impressive Herbs That Help Balance your Hormones. *Healthline.* Retrieved July 8, 2024, from https://www.healthline.com/nutrition/herbs-that-balance-hormones

29. Spritzler, F. (2021). 11 Natural Ways to Reduce Symptoms of Menopause. *Healthline.* Retrieved July 8, 2024, from https://www.healthline.com/nutrition/11-natural-menopause-tips

30. Engelmann, U., Walther, C., Bondarenko, B., Funk, P., & Schlafke, S. (2000). Extracts from fruits of saw palmetto (Sabal serrulata) and roots of stinging nettle (Urtica dioica): viable alternatives in the medical treatment of benign prostatic hyperplasia and associated lower urinary tracts symptoms. *Planta Medica, 66*(6), 557-563. https://pubmed.ncbi.nlm.nih.gov/11509966/

31. Hobbs, C. (n.d.). The Heart Herbs: Hawthorn and Garlic. *Christopher Hobbs's Library of Herbal Wisdom.* Retrieved July 8, 2024, from https://christopherhobbs.com/library/articles-on-herbs-and-health/the-heart-herbs-hawthorn-and-garlic/

32. Funk, J. L., Frye, J. B., Oyarzo, J. N., & Zhang, H. (2021). Synergistic Anti-Inflammatory Activity of Ginger and Turmeric. *Journal of Medicinal Food, 24*(1), 102-108. https://www.ncbi.nlm.nih.gov/pmc/articles/PMC9229778/

33. Zhou, J., Zhou, S., & Tang, J. (2000). Role of Fenugreek, Cinnamon, Curcuma longa, Berberine, and Their Derivatives in Insulin Resistance and Diabetes. *Therapeutic Advances in Endocrinology and Metabolism, 11*, 2042018820930906. https://www.ncbi.nlm.nih.gov/pmc/articles/PMC10145167/

34. The Herbal Academy. (n.d.). Choosing Safe Herbs for Your Kids. Retrieved July 8, 2024, from https://theherbalacademy.com/blog/choosing-safe-herbs-for-your-kids/

35. Mayway. (n.d.). Administering Herbs to Children. Retrieved July 8, 2024, from https://www.mayway.com/articles/administering-herbs-to-children

36. Rupa Health. (2021). Complementary and Integrative Medicine Treatment for Pediatric Sleep Disorders: Testing Supplements and Therapies. Retrieved July 8, 2024, from https://www.rupahealth.com/post/complementary-and-integrative-medicine-treatment-for-pediatric-sleep-disorders-testing-supplements-and-therapies

37. Jiang, Y., David, B., Tu, P., & Barbin, Y. (2020). Advancing herbal medicine: enhancing product quality and patient safety. *Journal of Ethnopharmacology, 250*, 112485. https://www.ncbi.nlm.nih.gov/pmc/articles/PMC10561302/

38. WHO Global Traditional Medicine Centre. (n.d.). *World Health Organization*. Retrieved July 8, 2024, from https://www.who.int/initiatives/who-global-traditional-medicine-centre

39. Denham, B. E. (2017). Athlete Information Sources About Dietary Supplements: A Review of Extant Research. *International Journal of Sport Nutrition and Exercise Metabolism, 27*(5), 470-483. https://doi.org/10.1123/ijsnem.2017-0050

40. Quantum Healing Pathways. (n.d.). Herbal Medicine: Mastering Dosage and Preparation Techniques. Retrieved July 8, 2024, from https://quantumhealingpathways.com/traditional-and-cultural-practices/ancient-medicinal-practices/exploring-herbal-medicine/understanding-the-dosage-and-preparation-methods-in-herbal-medicine/

41. Gouma, N. (n.d.). 5 Substances You Should Never Take While on Antidepressants. Retrieved July 8, 2024, from https://www.noragouma.com/5-substances-you-should-never-take-while-on-antidepressants/

42. Red Dragon Nutritionals. (n.d.). Exploring Saw Palmetto: Nature's Gift for Men's Health and Beyond. Retrieved July 8, 2024, from

https://www.reddragonnutritionals.com/blogs/news/exploring-saw-palmetto-natures-gift-for-mens-health-and-beyond

43. Supplement Sciences. (n.d.). The Maca Marvel: Enhancing Your Health with an Ancient Andean Root. Retrieved July 8, 2024, from https://supplement-sciences.nutriscape.net/maca/

44. Shoba, G., Joy, D., Joseph, T., Majeed, M., Rajendran, R., & Srinivas, P. S. (1998). Influence of piperine on the pharmacokinetics of curcumin in animals and human volunteers. *Planta Medica, 64*(4), 353-356. https://doi.org/10.1055/s-2006-957450

45. Lifestyle and Chronic Pain. (2022). Retrieved July 8, 2024, from https://doi.org/10.3390/books978-3-036

46. Golnoosh Torabian, Peter Valtchev, Qayyum Adil, Fariba Dehghani, Anti-influenza activity of elderberry (Sambucus nigra), Journal of Functional Foods. Retrieved July 26, 2024 from https://www.sciencedirect.com/science/article/pii/S1756464619300313

47. Kasper, S., Gastpar, M., Müller, W. E., Volz, H. P., Möller, H. J., Dienel, A., & Kieser, M. (2010). Lavender oil preparation Silexan is effective in generalized anxiety disorder—A randomized, double-blind, placebo-controlled trial. *International Journal of Neuropsychopharmacology, 13*(5), 633-641. Retrieved July 30, 2024 from https://doi.org/10.1017/S1461145709990943

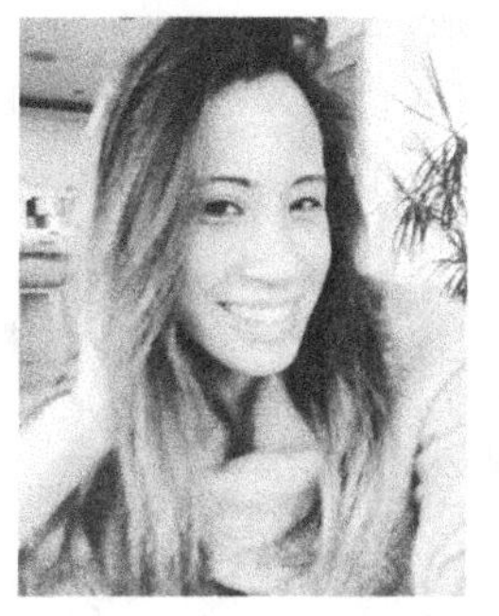

Sage Wilder is a passionate author and mum of two, dedicated to exploring the benefits of natural medicine and herbal remedies. Having spent several years immersed in holistic health, Sage champions using natural solutions to enhance wellness and manage health issues effectively. She is also a qualified yoga teacher with a degree in Biochemical Engineering and has delved into the study of Naturopathy.

Driven by a commitment to share her knowledge, Sage's mission is to demystify natural medicine and make it accessible to everyone, regardless of their background or experience. She aims to empower individuals to take control of their health using nature's resources, providing them with the tools needed for a healthier lifestyle.

Her enthusiasm for promoting healthier living through natural means is infectious, making her guides essential reading for those looking to adopt a more holistic approach to health. Sage continues to inspire and educate families on the importance of incorporating herbal and natural medicine into their everyday lives, ensuring long-term health and vitality.

* 9 7 9 8 3 3 5 9 9 7 9 4 2 *